Thriving or ł
Our lives with tw

of the cot

Richard Henry and Cath Lewis

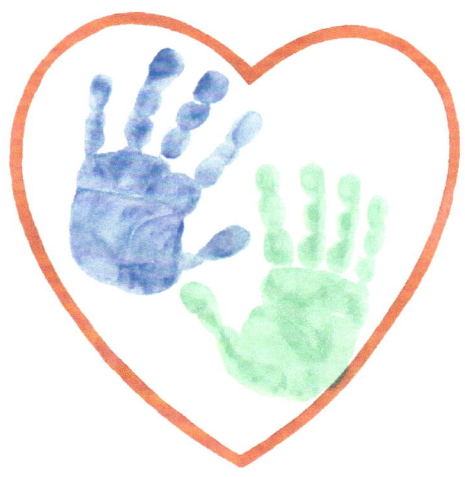

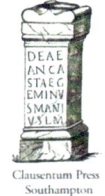

Clausentum Press
Southampton

First published in 2025 by The Clausentum Press

ISBN: 978-1-9192427-0-5
Published by Clausentum Press

A CIP catalogue record for this book is available from the British Library.

Printed in Great Britain

The images in this nook are minimalist watercolour interpretations of our own photographs

This book is a personal account of our experiences. It is not intended as medical or professional advice. Always consult a qualified health professional regarding any concerns about your own health or that of your child.

To the cousins Thomas, William, Peter, Lydia, Olivia and Evelyn for bringing the boys so much joy

Introduction

When we first started thinking about writing this book, it was because we couldn't find exactly what we were looking for. So many guides out there felt geared toward an American audience. We did not want to know about enormous cribs, colour-coded charts, and entire chapters devoted to insurance (because, sadly, they actually need that). Thank goodness for the NHS.

Otherwise the focus was on the "worst-case scenario" side of parenthood with multiples, leaving us more anxious than reassured. We felt a book could also be a bit comical, in the best possible way. Don't get us wrong: there are real risks, pregnancies can be complicated, and babies (especially twins) can test your patience in ways you never imagined. We certainly had our fair share of challenges along the way. But there is also joy, laughter, and, let's be honest, a lot of poo. We wanted a book that acknowledged all of it.

This book is part memoir, part practical guide. Sharing our story of the first year of the twins lives in a way that gives people an idea of what to expect, but also what might work for one family and what might not. Parenthood, particularly with twins, doesn't come with a one-size-fits-all manual. Sometimes the "tips" that look perfect on paper collapse spectacularly in the living room, along with the laundry pile. By sharing both our successes and our failures, we hope to offer something more real: a sense of how it feels, day to day, to navigate the highs, lows, and middle-of-the-night surprises.

We wrote it for anyone who might be facing a similar journey and wondering what it's actually like. There are no guarantees here. The twins might not sleep through the night, your toddler might throw their dinner at the cat, and yes, you will probably need more coffee than you thought humanly possible. But there is also wonder in the small moments. The kind of wonder that sneaks up when a baby grips your finger or their first smile. These moments can be chaotic, messy, often smelly, but they are also what make parenthood endlessly fascinating and worth every exhausting second.

Alongside our story, we've included tips, ideas, and reflections on what worked for us – and what didn't. This could be the routines that held us together, the tricks that saved us from tears (both theirs and ours), or the little rituals that became our family's own. None of it is perfect or guaranteed to work for anyone else, but we hope it gives readers a starting point, a bit of reassurance, and maybe a chuckle when they least expect it.

Ultimately, we wrote this book because we wanted to be honest. Honest about the messy, loud, joyful reality of raising twins and a sibling. The challenges we faced, and the support we received from friends, family, and our surprisingly opinionated chickens. It's a love letter to the chaos, the laughter, and the lessons learned along the way, and a guide for anyone stepping into this incredible, unpredictable journey to help feel just a little more prepared.

Honestly, without the NHS we would not have the twins, and maybe not even Cath. That is why we feel it is so important to give something back and support the amazing teams at the Princess Anne Hospital in Southampton who were there for us every step of the way. Every bit of profit we make from this book is going straight to the NHS to help them keep doing for others what they did for us.

Princess Anne Hospital is a major centre for multiple births. When we were there was only one double cot available outside of NICU. These cots make such a difference for families, keeping babies side by side just as they were in the womb, helping with bonding and comfort during those early, fragile days. We want to help families in Burley Ward in particular by donating all the profits from this book to help purchase much needed items. This may be a double cot or hospital grade breast pumps for example. The staff on the ward helped us get the best start for our journey we want to use this book to help them support other families with multiples on their wonderful journey.

If you would like to help even more, you can visit our fundraising page justgiving.com/crowdfunding/chrisandpaul We shall post updates every so often on how much the book has raised to date

About us, from three to five in a flash

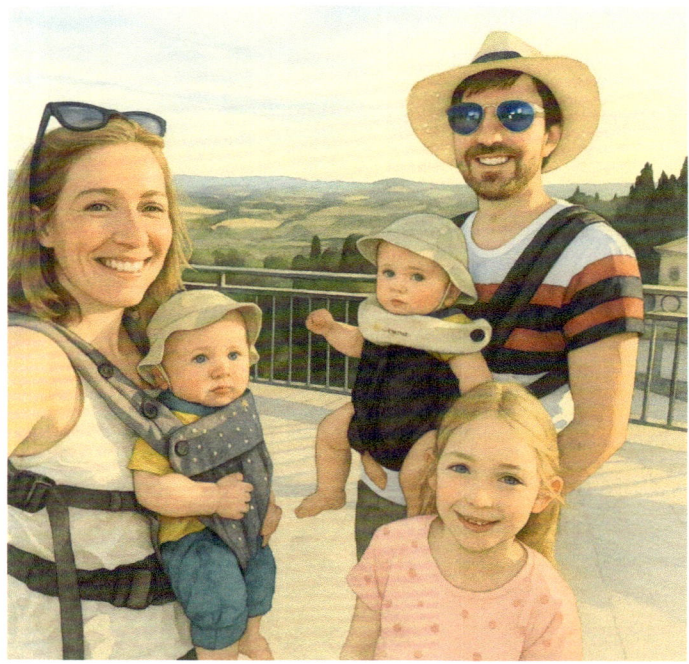

While our paths had crossed a few times through the usual six-degrees-of-separation type coincidences, Cath and I only properly started seeing each other in January 2020. Our first date is firmly lodged in my memory, though not necessarily for the reasons Cath intended. She'd suggested we go for a meal followed by a jazz night hosted by a friend of hers. Very civilised, very sophisticated.

Except… she got the date wrong. What we actually walked into was an open mic metal night, where half a dozen very enthusiastic but not especially tuneful singers took turns belting out Guns N' Roses. Imagine karaoke, but with extra distortion pedals and fewer inhibitions. Memorable, yes. Romantic?

debatable. After that, I gently suggested that I should perhaps take charge of planning future dates.

Still, when you find someone you connect with it feels like striking gold. Someone who shares your values, your sense of humour (even when it's about appallingly bad singing), and who you can sit with in the corner of a pub playing Jenga while quietly laughing at the world. Over the last five years we've been on quite a journey together. Cath, recently divorced when we met, has a wonderful daughter, Emma. It's been a joy watching her grow into such a confident, gregarious eight-year-old. Navigating all the ups and downs of the last few years as a family has had its challenges, but the constant has been the sense that we tackle them as a team.

I also remember that on our first date we ended up talking about the strange new virus spreading across the globe, a human version of a virus that Cath had researched in cats. At the time it still felt distant, but within weeks it would change everything. In March, just before lockdown I'd left my permanent role as a curator to take up what felt like a once-in-a-lifetime opportunity: joining the excavation of the Roman amphitheatre at Richborough in Kent. This was the very place where the Romans first landed in Britain, the sort of site archaeologists dream of. A dream opportunity that lasted precisely six days, at which point the first national lockdown hit and the project shut down. I'd taken a risk swapping stability for a short-term contract which evaporated almost immediately.

Like many people, I found the sudden shrinkage of the world disorientating. Overnight, my circle of contacts narrowed to almost no one. The constant rhythm of research, museums, and teaching just… stopped. Unlike most people, I also tried my best to avoid the dodgy Zoom quizzes, virtual pub nights and bake-offs that seemed to spring up overnight. In hindsight, that probably made my world even smaller and this certainly affected others detrimentally. I went into my shell, and it took a long time to come out again. Lockdown had its odd silver linings but it also pressed hard on the edges of who I thought I was. The year that started with metal karaoke leading to a new relationship, and a career high point instead turned into a masterclass in patience, resilience, and, if I'm honest, learning how not to lose my mind when every day looked exactly like the last, working on spreadsheets at home.

These days I'm back to being a curator of archaeology, after a few years spent researching the end of Roman Britain for my doctorate. My work looked at how, in the space of a generation, everything went tits up as the systems that had held society together simply unravelled. That's something we'd like to avoid repeating with the boys, though the circumstances today are rather different. In the fifth century you might have had to learn to wield a sword to adapt; today you can pick up a sideline through having woodworking instead.

Richard and I have written this book together documenting our experiences. It was also a period of change for me. A little while after discovering that I was going to become a single mum to a wonderful daughter, life took an unexpected turn. I decided to move back from Bristol to Southampton and moved in with my parents. It was a big change, but it worked surprisingly well for all of us; Nana, Papa, Emma, and me. We looked after each other in our own ways. Nana had been unwell with cancer for some time, but during her recovery we had plenty of lovely moments and memories which includes: Emma toddling along on walks with our cat Neo and loving sitting with him on a little bench as a toddler that is now perfect for the twins.

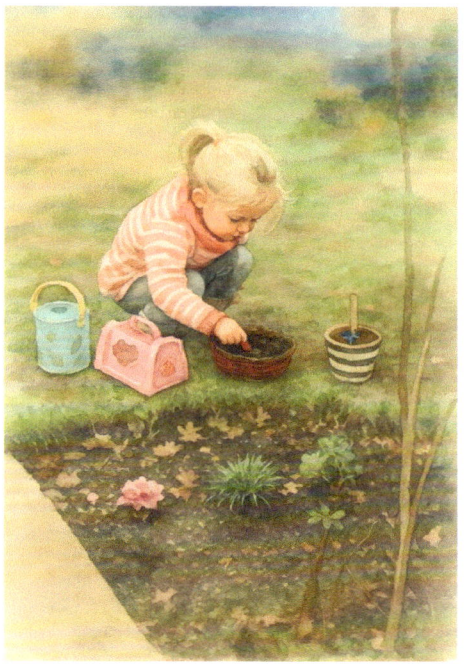

A few months after the global pandemic hit, Emma and I moved into what has since become our forever home. This slightly creaky but charming 1930s Collins house full of potential which had not been lived in for almost a decade. The 'secret' garden quickly became Emma's domain. She planted her very own bee garden and built a rather fancy bug mansion, which she took very seriously. Whenever we added an extra tack to the roof, she entertained herself by triumphantly exclaiming, "Nailed it!". Then repeating it after every single tack, "Nailed it!" … "Nailed it!" … "Nailed it!" The space is full of character, from the bee garden to the fairy village under the apple tree, complete with a resident fairy named Matilda who keeps a very close eye on things.

Somewhere in between gardening, fairy diplomacy, animal wrangling, and parenting, I (finally) finished my PhD studying the immune response to a chronic virus and returned to work as a vet. While there's less chance of being trampled on by a cow, life in first opinion small animal practice is never dull. One particularly memorable day involved all three vets, myself included, all trying to persuade a tortoise to bring his head out of his shell and open his mouth. We leaned in, coaxing and cajoling, offering gentle encouragement, only to be met with unwavering stubbornness. Eventually, we had to admit the tortoise had won, judging us all with the serene indifference only a tortoise can muster.

One thing people often say to us when they see us with the twins is, "You are doing so well and the boys are so cheerful". This is hilarious, because the reality is usually the opposite and one or the other has recently lost the plot! We think the only reason we've managed to give off this illusion is that we've got pretty good at being swans: calmish and serene above the surface, but underneath the water we're paddling away like we're in a two-man rowing final at the Olympics. Occasionally one of us forgets the stroke and drifts off sideways (usually towards coffee or gin) but somehow we always get back in sync.

Richard tells me it's a bit like being Sisyphus, endlessly rolling that big rock uphill. Except in our case the rock has wheels, one of which has fallen off, and the other is squeaking like mad. Just as you get it near the top of the hill, one twin decides to launch himself head-first off the side of the decking, while the other is howling because he's dropped the *only* spoon worth having (out of the twenty on the draining board). So down rolls the rock again.

But somehow, we keep pushing. If one of us is about to snap, the other usually finds a scrap of patience to step in. It's like we've developed this rhythm where one does the frantic paddling and rock-pushing while the other looks deceptively serene. That balance, that quiet teamwork with your soulmate, is probably the only reason we've ever managed to look like we're coping with life at all.

From the start, we've tried to keep our family values simple enough that even a toddler could (eventually) grasp them: be kind, be honest, look out for each other and laugh often. It has recently been extended to include no biting and no hair pulling. You would think 38 year-olds would behave better...

These values are not complicated, but it does make a difference. Most of our days are chaotic. There's shouting, spills, the odd toy launched at high velocity, a lot of poo, and sometimes a chicken pecking at the back door just to remind us who's really in charge. Underneath it all, the kids see that kindness gets remembered, honesty builds trust, and laughter gets us through. It does not always work, but we try to learn from our mistakes.

With more than one child, it's very easy for someone to get lost in the shuffle, especially with twins. They often get lumped together as "the boys." We've tried hard to make sure each child is seen as an individual, with their own quirks, favourites, and little victories. It means celebrating Paul's first steps as he applauds himself, or Chris finally not being terrified of his cuddly toy Zog, or Emma discovering she can balance Big Nige the chicken on her head.

It also means making sure Emma, as the big sister, never feels like she's just the "responsible older one," but gets her own space to shine. Sometimes that's as small as one-on-one story time, mounting her fantastic artwork, watching dance routines, or helping her with her latest elaborate den for the cats. The point is, no one should feel like they're just background noise.

We've found that talking about feelings openly, even when they're messy, illogical, or loud, makes the whole household run more smoothly. That goes for us adults as much as it does for the kids. If one of us is frazzled, saying so out loud is much better than pretending we're fine until the kettle explodes, something we do not always succeed with. With the kids, it means listening when they can't find the words but can certainly find the volume. Sometimes that communication is just "I don't want that spoon, I want the other spoon". But other times it's big stuff, like feeling left out, frustrated, or just needing a cuddle. A cuddle fixes a surprising number of problems.

It's often the kindness of friends and family that keeps everything running, whether it's the meal train after the twins were born, neighbours bringing round sourdough, or someone giving Cath five minutes of peace to attempt yoga. It rarely succeeds as Timmy the cat likes to attack anyone doing yoga and once any kids discover what they are doing the best-laid plans go awry!

It's tempting to wait for the big milestones. Be it first steps, first words or the first day at school. But some of the strongest connections come from the tiny rituals. Our made-up bedtime jokes that only we find funny. The completely ridiculous songs we invent while herding them into pyjamas, trying to eat their toes until they squirm giggling, or bribing the cats or chickens to sit still for a quick photo. The way we all laugh when the cat farts louder than the twins. Yes, Carter, we're looking at you. These small moments knit everything together. They're easy to miss in the chaos, but they're the glue that makes us a family, not just a group of people sharing a roof and a massive laundry pile.

Of course, we don't always get it right. Who does? What works one day doesn't always work the next. Especially with twins, an eight-year-old, as well as a clutch of small but mighty (and increasingly opinionated) chickens, two cats desperate for attention from anyone that does not grab their tails and a hampster. Reflecting on mistakes, laughing about them when we can, and adjusting as we go makes a big difference. Looking after two (sometimes three, or ten if you count the pets) takes a lot of work, but we generally balance things well as a team even if a wheel falls off now and then, or Feathers decides to roost on the outdoors dining table. It's definitely not picture-perfect, but it's consistent. And when the wheels do fall off, literally or metaphorically, we pick them up together and keep going. That's what makes this house feel like home.

Two peas one pod, finding out you are having twins

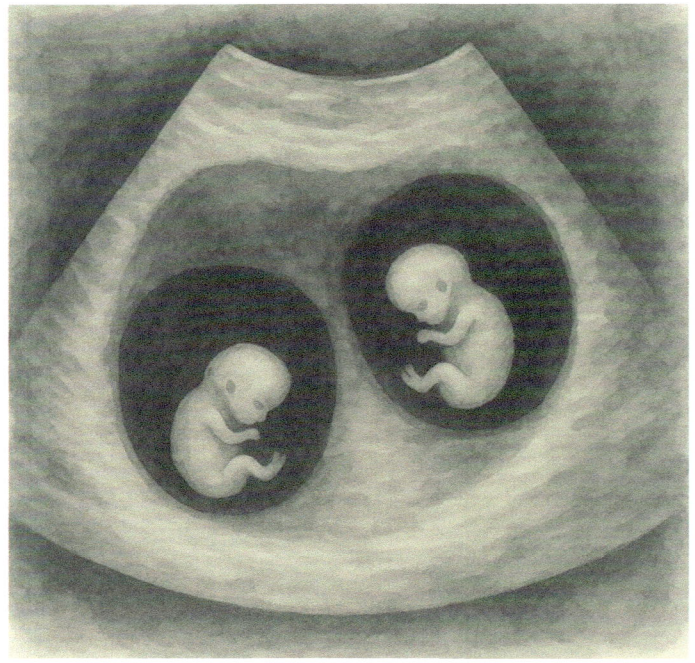

We first started talking seriously about having a baby in 2023. We were very conscious that this would mean the lives of our family, would change dramatically, especially Emma's as it always would for a first born. We wanted her to feel part of the adventure, not a bystander in someone else's story.

We found out we were expecting a baby in the last week of January 2024. We felt that rush of excitement you get when something you've been daydreaming about suddenly turns into a calendar entry. Even in those early days we had to tell a couple of people, not because we couldn't keep a secret, but because as a vet there are certain medicines and procedures that are very much on the "pregnancy no-no" list. If you are expecting you can't handle steroids, monoclonal antibodies (think of them as magic bullets directed against a particular protein), spray vaccines up a dog's nose, or inhale hamster anaesthetic for example.

Less than a week later, when I was about six weeks pregnant, I felt a searing pain on my right side near my hip/kidney. After speaking to my GP, we were sent for an ultrasound at the Princess Anne Hospital in Southampton. The concern was that the pregnancy might be ectopic. The reproductive equivalent of finding your house keys in the fridge; not where they're meant to be and potentially dangerous.

That scan will forever be one of the most unforgettable moments of our lives.

The trainee sonographer found an embryo measuring just 12 mm (about two-thirds the size of a 5p coin) located in the right place. We saw the tiny flicker of a heartbeat and breathed a sigh of relief. At the end of the scan she asked if we wanted a final look at the embryo and showed us a slightly different angle. But then she turned the screen away quickly, called over a colleague, and the two of them began whispering. Whispering is rarely good in medical settings, it's up there with "hmm" and "that's unusual". We sat there braced for bad news.

They showed us the embryo we'd already seen, confirmed its size and heartbeat, and we started to relax. Then they moved the scanner slightly to the right, and there it was: another faint flicker. A second embryo, smaller than the first. That was the moment we found out we were having twins.

We didn't get over the shock until the day they were born. Possibly not even then...

The size difference between them raised concerns. We were told there was a real chance the smaller twin might not survive the coming weeks. This is more common than people realise and many parents never even know it's happened. But we knew, and that made every scan a moment of suspense. We'd hold our breath until we saw two little heartbeats still flickering away.

At that stage, they couldn't tell what type of twins we had. Some types come with much greater risks, so we were booked to come back in two weeks. From that point onwards, the hospital became our second home. We were there either weekly or fortnightly until the birth and received exceptional care thanks to the wonderful NHS staff.

There are three main types of twins, and it all depends on when the fertilised egg splits. Here's a brief overview.

Dichorionic Diamniotic (DCDA): Two placentas, two amniotic sacs. These can be non-identical (fraternal) or identical twins who split very early. Least risky of the lot.

Monochorionic Diamniotic (MCDA): One placenta, two amniotic sacs. Always identical. They share a placenta but each has their own little bubble. This type is more closely monitored because of the risk of twin-to-twin transfusion syndrome (TTTS), where one twin hogs more blood than the other.

Monochorionic Monoamniotic (MCMA): One placenta, one amniotic sac. Rare and high risk because the babies can tangle their umbilical cords.

So yes, not just "help, we're having twins" but "help, what kind of twins are we having". The answer changes everything about your care. By week nine we found out they were identical MCDA twins. From then, they began to grow rapidly in our eyes, though they were still smaller than a singleton. The regular hospital trips were often a logistical headache, especially with work and childcare, but they were also a gift.

Normally, if you're carrying one baby and all is well, you have two scans: one at around 12 weeks and another at 20. We had scans fortnightly, sometimes weekly. Looking back, it was special. We knew the staff by name (or even their nicknames as we saw them so often). Every appointment could have brought bad news, but just as often it brought joy. Seeing them side by side, heartbeat by heartbeat, was extraordinary. And that's really what this book is about. Finding magic in the middle of the mayhem.

It was around this time we named the embryos Dave and Dave-Dave. No, we can't really explain why, but the names stuck. We could even spot their personalities before they were born watching them interact. Dave-Dave, the smaller one, was hitting Dave, who rolled away turning his back on his brother and started sucking his thumb in protest. The sacs are incredibly thin, imagine two babies inside balloons giving each other a poke. They could feel every movement through their very flimsy 'bedroom wall'.

In late March, a plastics warehouse near St Mary's Stadium in Southampton caught fire, just a few buildings away from the Archaeology Department where I work. The damage was huge, and for a while we were genuinely worried about our building. That day I rang Cath saying I was going to be back late and I spent the next few days going back and forth to assess the situation and protect what we could. Even the smoke could damage these irreplaceable objects.

It wouldn't surprise me if that smoke exposure led to what came next. Within a couple of weeks I was in A&E with pneumonia, having gone downhill fast in just 12 hours. Of course, typically it was the same day as our 20-week anomaly scan. Cath was nervous for many reasons, not least because a specialist had recently told her, "You're not really old, but in pregnancy terms, especially with MCDA twins, at 37 you are geriatric". A term that could have been delivered with a bit more finesse.

After treatment and 12 hours rest, I explained my situation to the A&E consultant, who grudgingly discharged me. A 10-minute walk took me almost an hour. I was overtaken by people with Zimmer frames who, by comparison, looked like they were in training for the Olympics. I was determined that I didn't want Cath to face the scan alone, especially if there was bad news. And, despite feeling like I had half a lung and the energy of a damp sponge, I made it.

Emotional reactions to having twins

There are a lot of different feelings you might have when you first find out you are expecting twins. Excitement, fear, disbelief, joy, sheer panic, mild nausea (possibly from the morning sickness, possibly from the news itself). Any of these are perfectly normal. In fact, if you can experience several of these in the space of a single afternoon, you are already training for the emotional gymnastics of parenthood.

Some people immediately start Googling "double pushchair best reviews" and "twins sleeping schedule" while others stare at the wall for three hours wondering if they've got enough mugs in the house for all the visitors who will turn up at once. Some do both. The important thing is this: whatever you feel, it's okay. There's no correct emotional response to learning you're about to double your family size in one go.

For us, the main question was: what on earth are we going to do? This was not an abstract question about parenting philosophy or whether we should try baby-led weaning. This was a very concrete, bricks-and-mortar problem. We have a modest three-bedroom house. There are already three of us. The maths is not complicated, but it is alarming.

After I had walked back to the car holding Cath's hand and cycled back to work I began mentally rearranging furniture in my head. Could we move someone into the garden shed? Not ideal. It has no central heating, and they would have to share the space with the lawnmower and the bandsaw. Could the twins share a cot until they were eighteen? Technically possible, but probably frowned upon.

When you find out you're having twins, practical questions such as these start popping up like uninvited relatives at Christmas. Where will they sleep? How will we fit two isofix car seats into the car? Actually, do we need a new car? Do we need a new house? Do we need new lives entirely? What the hell are we going to do?!

It's easy to feel overwhelmed, and in truth, we did. But we also found ourselves laughing at the absurdity of it. You can't plan for every possibility, and sometimes you have to lean into the ridiculousness of the situation. We regularly consoled ourselves that at least we weren't expecting triplets.

Twin pregnancy is not an everyday experience. In the UK, only about 1 in 65 pregnancies results in twins, which works out at roughly 11,000 twin births a year. Triplets and beyond? That's usually no more than 200 a year, basically enough to fill a decent-sized village hall, not much more. And within that, you've got all the variations. The rarer the set-up, the fewer people who've gone through exactly what you're experiencing. Making you part of a very small, very special club.

Here's another twist: while IVF and fertility treatments once drove up twin rates, the UK has drastically changed course. In the 1990s, about 28% of IVF pregnancies were twins. Thanks to a push for single embryo transfers, that rate fell to around 6% in 2019.

It helped to remember that countless parents have done this before us, many with less space and fewer resources. People make it work. Bedrooms get shared, furniture gets rearranged, the dining table becomes a nappy-changing station, and somehow life carries on. This book is a culmination of the frustration we felt because many books seemed to highlight the doom and gloom (not the dark humour and the fun that two tiny adventurers can bring),

The truth is, you probably won't have all the answers in those early days. That's fine. You don't need to have it all figured out before the babies arrive. In fact, you can't. Parenthood has a habit of ripping up your carefully prepared plans and replacing them with something entirely unexpected. Sometimes that's a challenge, sometimes it's a blessing, and often it's both at once.

What we wish we'd known in the early weeks of pregnancy

Your emotions will be all over the place: Excited one minute then googling "how many cots can you fit in a three-bedroom house" the next. Perfectly normal.

Early pregnancy symptoms can feel exaggerated with twins: You're not imagining it if you're exhausted after walking upstairs or if morning sickness is particularly awful.

Not every twinge is a disaster: But it's always worth getting checked, especially with twins. You will, however, develop an encyclopaedic knowledge of what your uterus is doing at any given moment.

Scans are more frequent and more nerve-wracking: The breath you hold before you see both heartbeats are still there could power a small wind farm. While this is terrifying, don't forget how special seeing them grow and interact truly is.

You'll get medical terms thrown at you early on: MCDA, DCDA, TTTS. You don't have to memorise them all at once; you'll have plenty of time to become fluent in Twin Abbreviations.

You will think about space. A lot: We don't mean the stars. Cupboard space, bedroom space, boot space in the car and the space in your changing bag… suddenly you are part parent, part budding estate agent. New specialist skills were rapidly developed, including compiling car boot volume comparison spread sheets… We probably should get out a bit more.

Naming them early is oddly comforting: Even if they're called "Dave" and "Dave-Dave" for now.

It's OK not to be glowing: You might be pale, tired, or green around the gills. That's also perfectly normal, despite what pregnancy magazines might suggest.

Looking back 18 months later, the hardest part was going into each scan not knowing if we would see a heartbeat for either Dave or Dave-Dave. Many people will know those nerves all too well. We were fortunate not to receive bad news, so we can't truly imagine the feelings of those who have, but we know how real that fear can be. Charities such as Tommy's and Sands provide vital support for anyone facing such uncertainty or loss.

Breaking the news (gently… sort of)

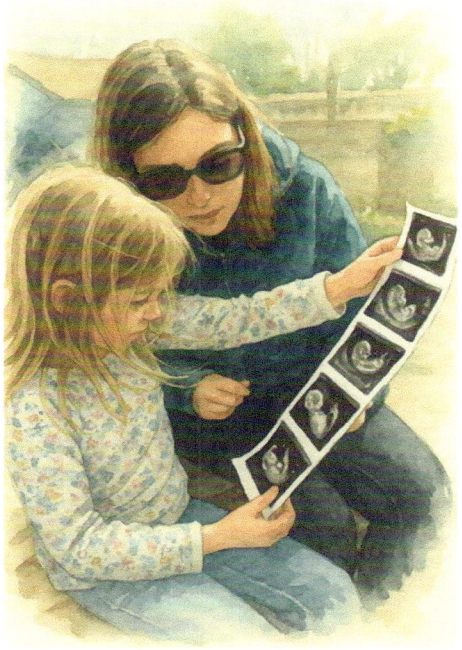

There were so many people we had to tell: Emma, friends and family. If we included every story of how we did it, this book would not be about twins but might serve better as a cure for insomnia. So, we've chosen just a few.

The first person we told was Cath's practice manager so she could help me covertly avoid certain procedures that might put the pregnancy at risk. I thought I was being very subtle at work but the whole team seemed to work it out within a couple of days (they all knew me too well).

A week later, we told Cath's cousins Helen and Martin, as their daughter Gina was getting married in a few weeks' time. I'd been invited to the hen do and didn't want to do any thunder stealing. With Helen's help, I attempted to blend in, armed with a few bottles of fizz, including some shockingly good alcohol-free stuff, and a large number of beige snacks. If anyone guessed, they were kind enough not to say, though I suspect my 'low-key' act wasn't quite as subtle as I thought and they deserve an Oscar pretending they hadn't noticed.

Whenever Richard told people we were having twins, he had a whole routine as it always took people by surprise. It started with, "Well, we went into hospital because we were worried it might be an ectopic pregnancy…". Then I'd describe the sonographer quietly showing us a tiny heartbeat, followed by a tense five-minute pause while they stared at the screen going "Hmm."

At this point in the story, most people would just nod politely, assuming it was going to end with "and everything was fine." That's when I'd drop the twist: the sonographer turned the screen again… and there was a second tiny heartbeat. The look on people's faces was pure gold, a mix of delight and confusion.

Only one person ever saw it coming: my colleague Emma. As soon as I reached the bit about the sonographer pausing, she just burst out laughing and said, "I know what you're about to say!" before laughing even harder. Honestly, it slightly ruined my punchline, but I forgave her, mostly because she was right. Emma also has twins, a boy and a girl. They even started walking on the very same day as each other, pausing long enough to give a wobbly high five and just about managing to stay upright. Perfect timing.

Telling family

It was the 13th of February when we decided to tell Richard's parents the news. We'd gone out for a lovely meal, and partway through I casually mentioned that I'd be starting a new job. Then I added that after an eight-month probation period, I'd be moving into an even bigger role. That's when we handed them the ultrasound pictures and the penny dropped. Not just a new job... two of them, arriving at the same time. They were, understandably, over the moon.

We didn't tell Cath's parents for another couple of weeks. By then, though, I was so exhausted that my dad began to suspect something was wrong, asking if I was okay, again, and again, and again. I just didn't seem myself. When we finally told them, Paul's reaction was, "Are you joking?" Perhaps he thought I was trialling an April Fools' prank early... and had really gone overboard with the props.

We only told my brothers a bit later on the phone while driving up to Gina's wedding. It was quite entertaining. The very first thing my brother Ed blurted out was, "Who's the father?" followed by, "What the hell have you done?" and then just laughter. Both of them couldn't quite tell if we were joking.

It was tricky keeping the news under wraps that day. We didn't want to steal anyone's thunder and only a couple of people knew at this point. Gina's sister Molly was probably the only one to clock it. Around 11:30pm she confronted me on the dance floor and said, "You're not telling me something. What's going on?" She kept repeating it, saying, "You've been holding that champagne for an hour and still haven't touched it. Spill it!". We thought we might be scuppered by this particular fizz as it was a very special one that was a favourite of my uncle Tom so she was right to be suspicious.

Telling Emma

We had spent a few weeks pondering how best to tell Emma but in the end, she clocked it anyway. One bedtime, as I was finishing a bedtime story, she looked at my tummy and said, "Mummy, are you pregnant?" I froze. It was not that I wanted to hide it from her, it was simply that 9pm on a school night was not the right time for such big news. I had no idea what to say so went with "I don't know," which was not exactly convincing but bought a little time.

Emma is incredibly special to both of us and we wanted her to be part of the excitement from the start. It was not just about telling her, it was about making her feel included in the story as it unfolded. I told her "You were right." and we put together a little envelope for her, tucking inside five ultrasound images. It was one of the first times she had seen a baby scan, and, as most people know, they are not always the easiest things to interpret.

We were all sitting outside and I pointed to one picture and explained, "This one shows a baby on the left… and if you look carefully, another one on the right." Emma's eyes widened, then narrowed as she studied the images. There were actually five pictures in total, some showing both twins, others close-ups. Emma looked again and asked, "Does that mean there are six babies?!" She looked genuinely alarmed. Fair enough! We would have been too if we had just been told we were having sextuplets.

Once the maths had been cleared up, she was delighted. A few days later, at another scan, we told the sonographer how Emma had taken the photos into school for show and tell. From that day on, she often printed an extra copy just for Emma, so she could take a fresh one to class each time. It was a small gesture, but it meant the world to her. The staff made all of us feel part of the process, not just me.

On 1st May 2024, the Dave and Dave-Dave "wrote" Emma a letter. It said:

"We are 17 weeks today, and we're so excited to meet you! On our last scan, we were practically dancing with excitement. It'll be a few more months until we're born, but until then, you can call us Dave and Dave-Dave, the twins."

Emma looked at us seriously and wailed, "I lost the bet!".

"With who?" we asked.

"You!" she shot back.

At this point, Emma was really hoping for girls. But looking back, if you're eight years old and suddenly you have twin sisters who gang up on you and steal all your stuff, you'd probably be pretty frustrated. Luckily, with Paul and Chris adoring her every move, she's got a very dribbly, dedicated (until they spot a strawberry) little army on her side!

When Dave and Dave-Dave gave us multiple scares

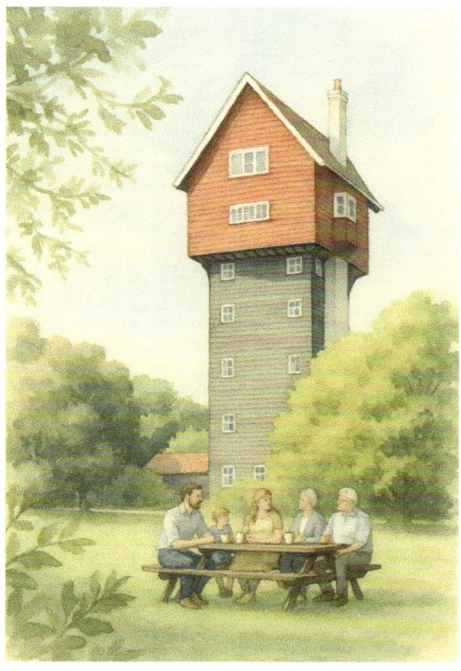

By week 20, things started to get complicated. In MCDA twin pregnancies like ours, one of the most important checks is the fluid level around each foetus. These "amniotic fluid pockets" are measured to ensure both foetuses are sharing resources fairly. Consistency is good. Sudden imbalance is not.

An imbalance can signal TTTS, where one twin receives too much blood and the other too little. In one scan, the measurements shifted dramatically: Dave suddenly had far more fluid than Dave-Dave, and the change had happened in just days. TTTS can develop frighteningly fast, and before 23 weeks, the prognosis is grim.

I had just had Covid and it seems inflammation caused by my immune response to the virus triggered this imbalance. It was a nerve-wracking time, every scan felt like an exam we might fail. From then on, we were seen weekly until given the all clear. Once we reached week 23, we brought a hospital bag to every appointment in case we had to go straight to surgery or delivery. We started taking life one day at a time with every week the twins stayed *in utero* becoming a little cause for celebration.

Eighteen months earlier, Richard's parents had booked a once-in-a-lifetime family stay at The House in the Clouds in Thorpeness, Suffolk. A five-storey converted water tower with panoramic views and over seventy stairs. No lift. Amazing if you are agile, less so if heavily pregnant with twins, iron-deficient, and short of breath. We stayed in the lowest bedroom to minimise climbs, but even that was exhausting as it was still three stories up.

During the week, my breathing worsened, and after experiencing chest pains, I checked in with the midwives in Southampton and they advised me to go straight to A&E to be checked over, arriving in Ipswich just after midnight. Richard had been socialising with his family and godfather, so he couldn't drive for a little while, but he stayed with me. At 6am he went back to explain things to Emma so she wouldn't wake to find her mum gone and panic. Emma spent the day with my parents and Bob and Tina exploring Thorpeness while Richard returned to the hospital.

I had not slept and was emotionally drained. I was sat next to a man loudly coughing with Covid yet determined to only half wear a mask, while a woman with dementia was strolling around the wards gleefully set off every alarm she could reach. Amid this chaos for Cath, Richard returned armed with a fancy salmon bagel from The Three Magpies Bakery, a San Pellegrino and a hug. It is the little things that help.

The consultant suspected a pulmonary embolism, a blood clot in the lungs, which required scans to diagnose, but also the worry of radiation exposure during pregnancy. I understood the implications, and Richard watched me asking detailed questions, not fully realising the seriousness of some of the tests. He could tell by my face that I was uneasy about the potential impact from radiation on Dave and Dave-Dave. We avoid Google; otherwise, we might conclude that nappy rash is a rare flesh-eating disease. Only later did we truly appreciated the gravity. For 4 in 100 pregnant women who experience pulmonary embolism, it is fatal.

To mitigate the risk of a clot, I was shown how to inject myself just under the skin, a task far easier in animals than humans. A few days later, we returned for a ventilation-perfusion scan, a procedure that confirmed no clot and no acute concerns. Thankfully my precautionary treatment was stopped. We returned to our holiday relieved but renewed in our appreciation of how physically and emotionally draining a multiple pregnancy can be.

When we left the house in the clouds, we detoured back to the AMSDEC ward at Ipswich Hospital who had looked after me. Emma had drawn a picture for the staff and wanted to take some chocolates to say thank you for looking after me. Unfortunately, the department was closed, which was a bit of a disappointment. Emma's perfectly timed gesture met with locked doors. But then, as we were leaving, by chance we bumped into one of the people who had cared for me. Emma was able to hand over the picture and chocolates in person.

It was clearly a surprise for him too, he was visibly moved, even tearing up slightly. Emma's gratitude was clear to see, her mum and unborn brothers had faced a very real risk from a blood clot, so this simple gesture felt huge. It was a little reminder of how brilliant the NHS can be, even if timing sometimes works against you. And, of course, Emma got to feel like a tiny superhero for the day.

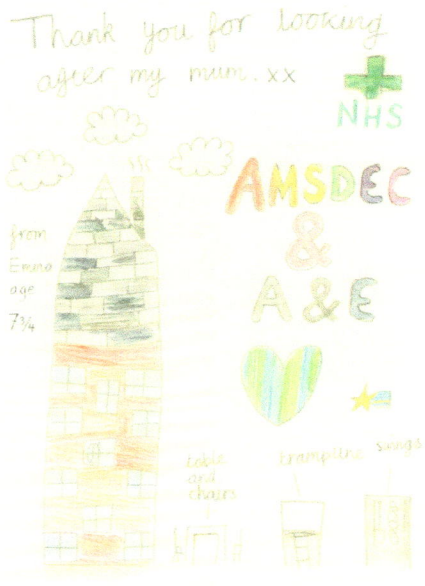

The following weekend, we went to see friends of ours, Alan, and his wife Rachel who Richard knew from when he worked in Salisbury. Alan, more than anyone else, has helped us prepare for family life in practical ways. He taught me woodworking, helped me build both an office and a workshop, and even lent a hand with our fence. Given that he lives an hour and a half away, we're incredibly lucky that he's so generous with his time; without him, I honestly don't know how we would have managed.

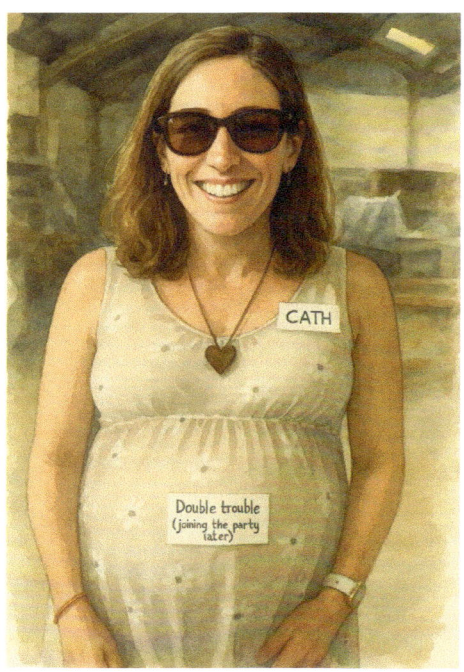

Alan always makes us laugh. For the last few years, he's been restoring a series of magical waterfalls on the estate he works for with a dedicated group of volunteers. He had invited us to join his family BBQ. Given he was one of seven, many of whom have two or three children of their own, it was a huge event. He has 15 nieces and nephews who have 18 kids themselves. With so many people, name badges were essential: one for Cath, one for Emma, one for me, and (crucially) one for the bump, labelled "Double Trouble, joining the party later."

While we tried to remain light-hearted and relaxed, that summer remained tense with the looming possibility of TTTS. Each weekly scan carried the potential for devastating news. We tackled it week by week: every milestone, 23 weeks, 26, 30, 36, was a victory. These extra days inside the womb significantly improve a twin's health and development.

Here's how the weeks translated into their growth:

Week 23: About the size of a large mango. Practising breathing movements, but not yet ready for life outside the womb. Survival in neonatal units is possible but highly risky.

Week 26: Lungs developing tiny air sacs and producing surfactant. Eyes opening, responsive to sound. Likelihood of survival improves but intensive support still needed.

Week 30: Around three pounds each. More fat, better brain and lung development. Weeks in neonatal intensive care expected, but outlook is better.

Week 32: Rounder faces, smoother skin. Most can breathe without help or minimal support. Digestive systems developing; tube feeding may be needed. Risks of major complications lower.

Week 36: Late preterm, recommended induction for MCDA twins (37 weeks for fraternal twins). Usually 5–6 pounds, mature lungs, can feed, breathe, and regulate temperature independently. Most go straight to the postnatal ward.

In August, we went to the hospital because I was starting to have contractions, and, as you can probably imagine, it scared the living daylight out of us. They were strong, irregular, and worrying enough to make it look like things might happen straight away. In reality, they were a precursor called Braxton Hicks contractions. It seems pregnancy with multiples in general have a particular flair for giving false alarms.

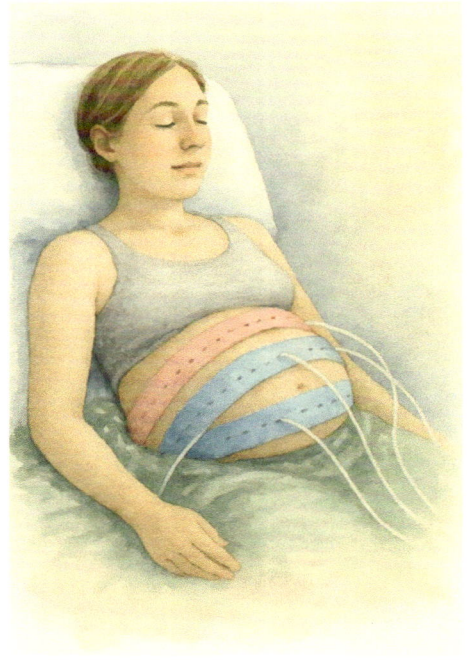

It was on this trip that I met my nemesis, the cardiotocography (CTG) machine. A staple of late multiple pregnancies, it tracks babies' heartbeats and maternal uterine contractions. For twins, three sensors are strapped to your bump, two monitor heart rates via Doppler ultrasound, the other measures uterine tightening. The results appear as wiggly lines on paper: one for each baby and one for contractions. Patterns are studied for steady heart rates, movement responses, and reactions to contractions.

It's not as simple as it sounds. Distinguishing between two heartbeats, or one repeated, requires copious gel, frequent repositioning, and endless patience. The straps themselves intensified contractions and caused immense pain, made even worse because I wasn't allowed to move. Imagine trying to keep still while strapped into a CTG machine, your bump smeared in gel, and every little jolt sending shocks of pain through you. It's a bit like being a Christmas turkey that's somehow developed Braxton Hicks.

We'd been trying to book little escapes all summer, every week, every day, even with the constant worry of a twin-to-twin transfusion and early birth hanging over us. So, we were really looking forward to a relaxing day at Reading Lido after Cath went on maternity leave. Only to discover that you can't enter with a car over 2 m high and we had a roof box. Cue mild panic: With Cath in the car, I had to figure out how to get it into a different car park when it barely fit through that barrier as well. After some delicate manoeuvring, I just about wedged the 500 litre roof box into the car. It was a very close squeeze and left little room for the driver.

We had a lovely lunch and then went for a massage. Unfortunately, I turned out to be allergic to something in the massage oil and my face swelled up like I'd had a kilogram of lip filler in each lip. With me looking like a human balloon, Cath had to waddle off to Tesco alone to fetch some Piriton to bring the swelling down. Once we were finally ready to leave, I had the joy of getting the rooftop box back on the roof while looking like an inflated balloon.

When rolling over becomes an Olympic sport: Pregnancy with twins

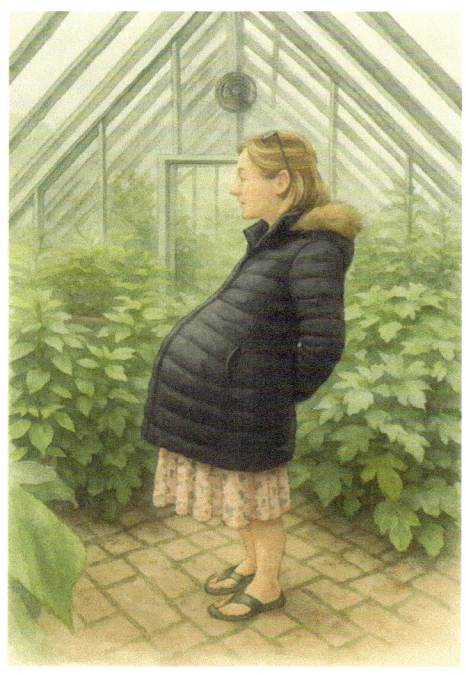

We found out very early that we were expecting twins, so by six weeks I already knew there were two little foetuses draining my energy and not just one. At least I had an explanation for why I felt so rough. Some of it was probably down to being nearly a decade older than when I was pregnant with Emma, and some of it was working in a busy vet clinic on my feet all day, wrangling pets of varied size and temperament. It was a very different experience to my previous pregnancy where I worked in the lab, where the only thing I had to lift was a multichannel pipette. The nausea and fatigue were on another level compared to my singleton pregnancy.

Last time, I could finish work and collapse on the sofa, but this time we had a seven-year-old waiting at home. There was no chance of putting my feet up with after-school activities, spellings, homework, dinner, bath, and bedtime routines to get through first. It felt like having two jobs, except one of them involved being repeatedly corrected on Year 3 spellings by someone under four foot tall (usually they were wrong). By the end of the day I was often asleep in her bed, book still in hand, having conked out halfway through Harry Potter long before she did.

I did not have cravings as such, but I did develop a strong preference for beige food rather than the healthier options I would normally go for. Quinoa was firmly out, crisps were in. For anyone who knows me, that was unusual enough to raise eyebrows. Eating was the only thing that eased the morning sickness, so the car became a snack haven, with bags of nuts and other treats stashed in the glove box and door compartments. My consulting room cupboard quickly became a secret tuck shop too. My colleagues were brilliant, regularly sneaking in drinks, biscuits, or anything else to keep me going, and trying their best to build breaks into my hectic days.

Even so, I got so big so quickly that examining dogs became a logistical challenge. I often ended up sitting cross-legged on the floor with them, because bending was too uncomfortable and hoisting them onto the table was out of the question.

One thing that did take me by surprise was that I became jumpy around dogs barking. I did not feel nervous, but my reflexes had reset themselves to high alert, like some internal bodyguard had been installed to protect Dave and Dave-Dave.

In the long run, just getting out of the car became its own challenge. Princess Anne is a maternity hospital with the smallest car parking spaces imaginable, and we often saw heavily pregnant women struggling to squeeze themselves out of the doors, myself included. Honestly, it felt less like antenatal care and more like qualifying heats for some kind of Olympic gymnastics event. By 30 weeks I was already much bigger than I had been at term with Emma. We tried all sorts to help me stay comfortable, from maternity belly bands to several pregnancy pillows, but there was no ignoring the sheer weight pressing down on my skeleton. It was the equivalent of carrying an 11 lb baby plus all the bonus features, strapped to me like a badly packed rucksack.

One day I felt so dreadful I barely made it into work before admitting defeat. My wonderful manager insisted I lie down on the staff sofa while Richard cycled over from his job to pick me up. Thank goodness the fantastic Princess Anne Hospital was only half a mile away, because even that short trip felt like a marathon. One of the staff we got to know well walked me down to the right department while Richard parked the car, a kindness I'll always remember.

The care I received was exceptional. Our consultant and two specialist midwives were calm, consistent, kind (or brutally honest when needed, telling me to rest and "behave"). But the pregnancy was taking a toll. My iron levels had crashed. The twins were hoarding all my reserves: biologically impressive, physically miserable. For weeks, I had been taking over-the-counter iron supplements (25mg), which the consultant dismissed as "Smarties," and switched me to 200mg tablets. Effective, yes. Gentle on the stomach, no.

Normally, I am a whirlwind, the sort of person who can work a full day, reorganise a cupboard, and still find the energy to paint the shed. Now, climbing the stairs felt like Mount Everest. The consultant described me as "as pale as the grey blind" and firmly told me to rest. Naturally, I carried on working another week until finally agreeing to be signed off only a little begrudgingly.

All through the pregnancy we were lucky to have two specialist midwives who became our lifeline. One of them, in particular, was far more than a healthcare professional. She was a steady, reassuring presence in the middle of chaos. She celebrated every little milestone with us, answered endless questions without judgment, and always seemed to know when we needed an extra bit of encouragement. She even visited us several times, both while we were waiting for induction and again after the boys arrived. Meeting her while holding Chris and Paul felt like a full-circle moment. We could finally show her what all those months of care and kindness had helped us achieve.

To say thank you, Richard made little stars for her, for the sonographer we saw most, and for the member of staff who looked after me when I was very unwell and walked me from the foetal medicine unit to the day unit downstairs. He made them Christmas decorations from an unusual ash burr. Ash is said to symbolise protection, which felt fitting. The wood had beautiful, intricate patterns, and turning it into something personal was the least we could do to show our gratitude. A small gesture, perhaps, but one that mattered deeply to us. It was our way of giving back to the team who had carried us through those months and helped bring our boys safely into the world.

The big arrival: labour, birth, and the unexpected

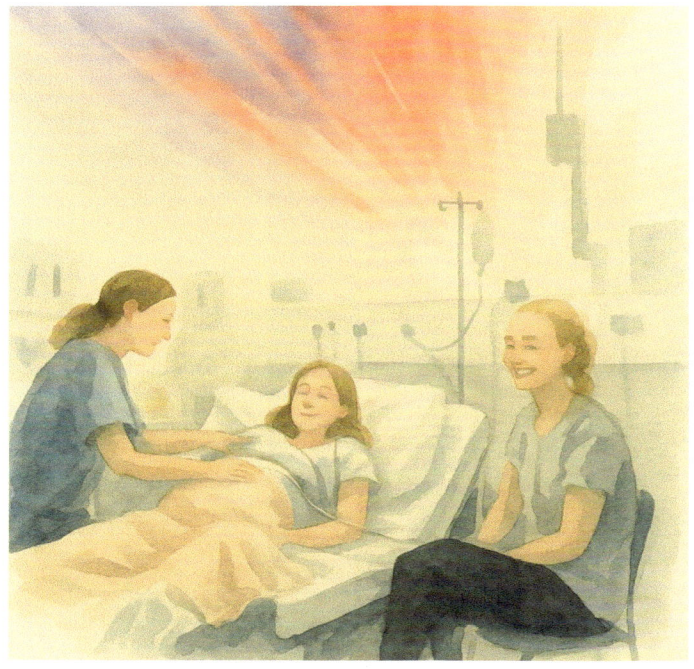

When we first spoke to the consultant about booking the date for induction, she suggested the 9th of September which just so happens to be Cath's birthday. That seemed a bit unfair! Imagine spending your birthday with a disappointing type of balloon only given to special people for inductions. We were grateful when it was moved to the 10th.

To mark the occasion, Cath, her parents, and I went to The Pig in Brockenhurst for a special meal, since we didn't think we'd have the chance to go out again anytime soon. Throughout the meal, Cath looked a little uncomfortable, probably wondering if the babies might decide to arrive mid-Orangery or worse, mid meal. Luckily for everyone, double trouble made no surprise guest appearance.

The next day, on arrival at the hospital, staff shortages meant everything was delayed. The induction began with a prostaglandin tablet to soften the cervix, the first step in what was going to be a long day. Labour ward waiting areas are a strange mix of coexisting emotions: empathy and exhaustion, hope and despair. I remember one partner in tears from the pain while her other half was busy calling energy companies to compare rates. And then there was the woman who hadn't eaten for more than 24 hours because she was waiting for an epidural, while the father-to-be happily ate a bucket of KFC by her bedside. Safe to say, don't provoke a woman in labour. You might think you can run away, but she won't forget.

NHS guidance offers different induction methods:

- low-dose prostaglandin tablets (vaginally)
- Prostin pessaries
- Foley balloon catheters
- oxytocin drips

The chosen method is based on cervical readiness and staffing. After 12 hours, the tablet hadn't done enough. A second vaginal exam was promising enough to break my waters based on a Bishop score (A cervix readiness score predicting labour or induction success; 8 or more is favourable), but there was no room yet. We waited again while staff and space became available. We even discussed the Foley balloon catheter which is a small, fluid-filled balloon that dilates the cervix naturally. Eventually, a wonderful midwife and a room became available, and the process could finally begin. Unfortunately for us, the

Bishop score was much lower than 8 so the planned breaking of the waters was called off at the last minute.

Throughout, Cath was strapped to her nemesis, the CTG machine, for hours at a time. Luckily, we had a mobile monitor for a while, which let me move around and reduced discomfort during contractions.

We had to wait another day (the third in hospital) but once the waters were broken the birth quickly proved to be… let's say "full-on." Machines went ping like a budget hospital remix of *The Magic Roundabout*. Cath was in considerable pain and asked for an epidural, which made a world of difference. Her contractions lasted far longer than average. Normally you would expect three in ten minutes, hers stretched to 90–120 seconds a time. Five hours in, a shift change brought in a new pair of midwives. Around this time, I noticed something strange. Cath's bump, which had been enormous, suddenly looked like half of it had disappeared. At the same moment, one of the heartbeats vanished from the monitor.

A mobile ultrasound scanner revealed the culprit. Once the waters broke, Dave-Dave had gone on his first of many adventures moving into a transverse position to say hi to his brother before becoming breech. Dave-Dave's first adventure may also have been the cause of the prolonged contractions.

What had been a gentle jog became a full sprint. Within 10–15 minutes, we moved from the calm of the birthing room to the bright lights of the theatre. The theatre was packed: at least two consultants, several midwives, and what felt like a small football crowd, each with a role. Incubators and equipment were ready. The NHS's efficiency, organisation, and kindness were on full display. We were lucky to have a wonderful anaesthetist attending to Cath who had the most amazing surgical cap with the solar system and rockets on it.

This stage was particularly tricky for Cath. We arrived at the theatre an hour before the boys finally made an appearance. Paul had been lodged in the same position since around week 15 or 16, with his head wedged against Cath's pelvis - like an overstuffed sofa in a too-small doorway. Despite best efforts, he wouldn't budge. If a episiotomy and forceps were not successful we would require an emergency caesarean. Cath's epidural was topped up (making pushing a real challenge) and the surgery team started scrubbing up in preparation. With a lot of skill (and some physics-defying manoeuvres), Paul finally made his entrance at 11.15pm, weighing 5lb 10oz.

Dave-Dave added extra drama. Facing the wrong way, he set off on his second adventure and tried to swim off in entirely the wrong direction. Several midwives pressed on Cath's abdomen to keep him in place while the doctor worked. Several attempts were made to catch him by his ankles and his feet slipped away each time. We were told after one final attempt it would need to be an emergency caesarean. Luckily, this one final try was successful and Chris was pulled out by his feet. He cried immediately, then suddenly stopped. That pause is the longest a parent will ever hear. Cath knew something was wrong. The team acted fast, resuscitating him, and moments later he was breathing again. Chris was born at 11.23pm and weighed 5lb.

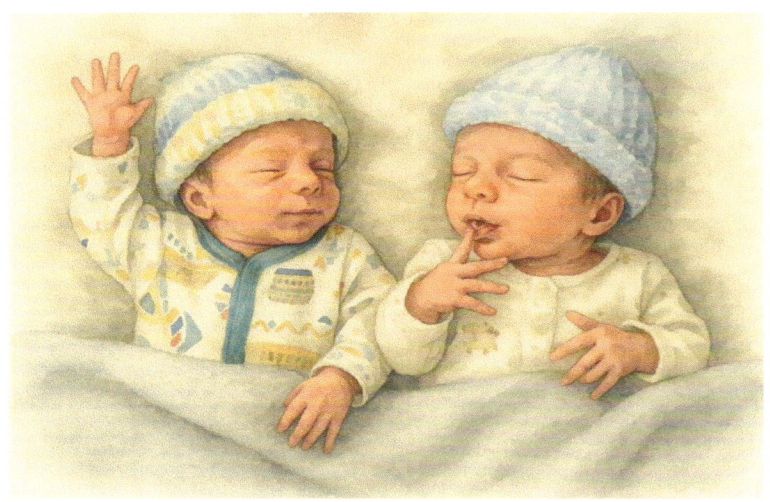

In the final stages, the midwives were tickled by our embryo names. Three midwives were firmly pushing on Cath's abdomen, gleefully shouting, "Come on Dave-Dave! Come on Dave-Dave!" Meanwhile, other staff looked on, baffled. Later, one midwife confessed she was thoroughly entertained, especially when colleagues asked her if we were seriously naming the babies Dave and Dave-Dave. The midwife stared them down deadpan: "Yes, they are." Their response: "Oh…"

And just like that, we had two tiny, perfect boys. Slightly dishevelled, definitely dramatic, but absolutely ours. Both boys were incredibly small, the tiniest babies Richard had ever seen, and surprisingly hairy. Miniature wolverines complete with soft, downy fur especially on their ears and shoulders. Apparently, this hair usually disappears by 35–36 weeks, but for now, they could easily star in a BBC nature documentary.

The fold-out bed provided for partners was broken, and my grumblings were clearly annoying Cath so she thought me getting a proper night's sleep was more sensible and she and the midwives persuaded me to go home. I managed a few jobs, grabbed clean clothes, and restocked supplies as our planned hospital stay had already eaten into our packed bags.

That night while Richard was at home, I was struggling to move properly because of the lingering effects of the epidural. Dave (the last time he'd be called that) took advantage, peeing directly on his own face and all over both of us during his very first nappy change. Equal parts tragic and hilarious.

By the time I got back to the hospital Cath and the boys had moved from the labour ward to a post-natal ward. I took over so that she could get some much needed rest. Then, out of nowhere, Cath sat bolt upright in bed, panic in her voice: "Where are they!? Where are they!?" She was absolutely convinced that we had four babies, not two, and that somehow three of them had gone missing because Chris was being checked over. It took a few frantic moments, and a lot of reassurance, before she accepted that we were, in fact, only responsible for two very real, very tiny humans. Sleep deprivation does strange things to you.

NICU, Birth, and Early Arrivals

Having twins means you learn quickly that birth plans are more like… guidelines. Early arrivals are pretty common, and with twins, "term" often comes a little sooner than expected. With MCDA twins for example term is 36 weeks because the placenta has ran two marathons by this point. That means feeding challenges, jaundice and a stint in the NICU might be on the cards.

Ah, the NICU. Neonatal Intensive Care Unit. Sounds intimidating, doesn't it? And it is… at first. Lights are bright, monitors beep in every direction, and tiny babies lie hooked up to more wires than a spaceship. It was strange seeing our two boys lying there in an incubator but luckily for us this did not last long. Even a short NICU stay would be an intense education in multitasking, patience, and learning how to love someone through a sea of beeping machines.

Birth Methods: Vaginal vs. C-Section

Twin births are unpredictable. A few parents breeze through natural vaginal births. Others end up in the operating theatre, caesareans in progress, feeling simultaneously grateful and stunned. Planned c-sections bring some predictability, but nothing quite prepares you for the surreal moment when two babies appear in less than ten minutes, or for the fact that you then have to recover from major abdominal surgery while caring for two tiny humans.

Recovery after a vaginal birth brings soreness, leaking, and all the usual "you'll feel like you've been run over by a small truck" moments. It will take longer if other methods such as forceps are used.

Recovery after a c-section adds multiple layers of stitches, limited mobility for six weeks, and the daily challenge of not bending, lifting, and reaching while carrying an extra-special cargo, your twins. Expect every move to feel like a mini workout, every feed an Olympic event, and every nappy change a tactical mission.

Recovery with Multiples

Recovering from giving birth to twins is like doing three marathons you knew were coming up but couldn't train for, having to do it blindfolded while juggling. Sleep becomes a distant memory, feeding is constant, and "me time" is practically a myth. Even when both babies nap at the same time, a rare and magical event (at least for us), you'll probably spend that time staring at the ceiling, wondering how anyone survives this phase. In the first few days self-care involves luxuries such as being able to brush your teeth and if you are very lucky even have a shower.

Support is essential. Partners, friends, and family can help with meals, laundry, or simply holding a baby so you can shower without guilt. Recovery is not just about your body, it's about surviving the emotional rollercoaster, which can include anxiety, mood swings, and the occasional panic about whether either twin is getting enough milk. Some babies, especially if they arrive prematurely, may also face health challenges such as jaundice or other early difficulties. These are very common and treatable but can add to the worry. We found the key to survival was accepting that some days will be messy as well as smelly, and every day in the beginning is chaotic with twins.

The first few days

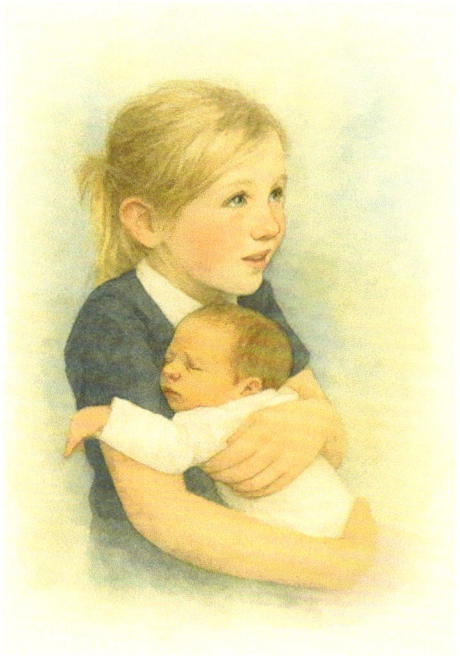

A few days after the babies were born, Richard's mum and dad went to collect this absolutely amazing second hand feeding cushion that really helped us out in those early months. It even had little pigs on it, quite cute, really. We figured it was the perfect time to introduce the grandparents to the twins names when they dropped it off.

I think mum had an inkling of what we were about to do, I might've slightly given it away when she'd asked previously. Dad, on the other hand, had absolutely no idea.

We have a lovely little video of mum holding Paul and saying, "Mum, this is Paul Henry," and then dad holding Chris and us saying, "Dad, this is Chris Henry." dad genuinely looked very touched. Mum, meanwhile, looked slightly offended and asked why neither of them was called Alison, which I thought was fair enough, but let's be honest, that only really works if you're called Sue.

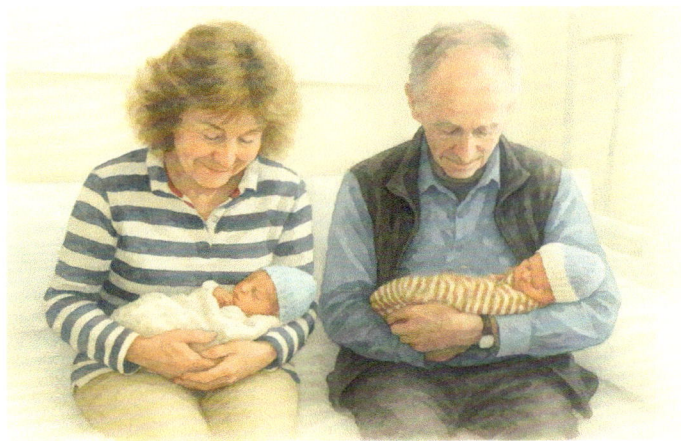

Then it was Cath's turn with her parents. "This is Chris Henry," she said to her mum Sue, who was very excited. When we introduced Paul to Paul he looked a bit shocked and his first reaction was, "Are you sure you want to do that?". We're not entirely convinced he thought it was a good idea, but both of our fathers are both lovely people and very important role models in our lives.

Of course, before we got to that fun bit, there were the routine newborn checks. In those first few days, babies in UK hospitals are treated like tiny, delicate celebrities on a round-the-clock reality show. Every few hours, someone would come along to check their temperature and measure their heart rate. There were also weight checks and checks to make sure all the necessary body parts were present and functioning. A visual checklist was essentially "two arms, two legs, one nose, ten fingers, ten toes, and please, please, no surprise extra organs."

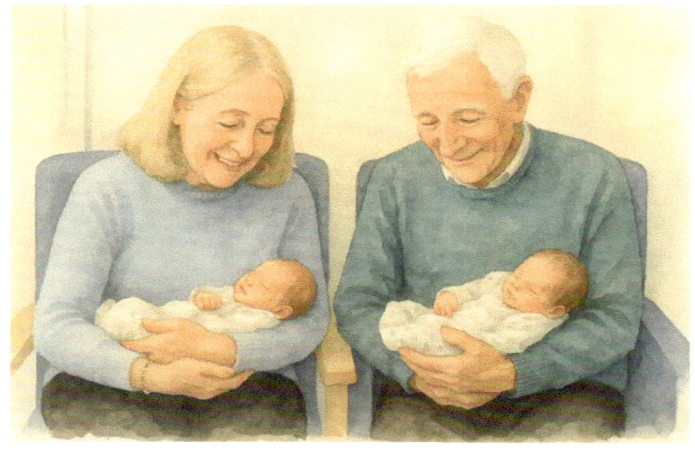

Then came the infamous heel prick tests. This is when a nurse pokes the baby's heel to collect a few drops of blood. To the babies this probably felt like being ambushed by a tiny vampire. That blood would be tested for a range of conditions, from rare metabolic disorders to cystic fibrosis. The nurses always handled it with incredible care, but for parents, it was nerve-wracking watching their tiny humans go through what felt like a torturous process. Paul, in particular, ended up with pin cushions for heels by the end of our stay.

Alongside that, there were all the other checks: hearing tests, eye screenings for cataracts, weight and feeding monitoring. The frequency of these checks meant we were essentially living in a cycle of feeding, measuring, testing, changing nappies, and trying to catch a minute of sleep somewhere in between. It was exhausting, but it did make the boys look like they had tiny personal assistants dedicated solely to their well-being. We were happy to have those assistants, even if they did arrive every three hours like clockwork.

Both boys, like the vast majority of twins, developed jaundice, a yellowing of the skin that's very common in newborns particularly if preterm. It happens because their livers are still maturing and can't yet process bilirubin properly. Most of the time it clears up on its own, but sometimes treatment (light therapy) is needed to help things along. It can look alarming, but with proper monitoring and intervention if needed it's rarely dangerous. Apparently, having two in the womb can mean your liver is a little slower to get its act together when they are also preterm and tend to be smaller. We were told not to worry too much, but seeing the yellow tinge creeping across their skin definitely made us pay attention.

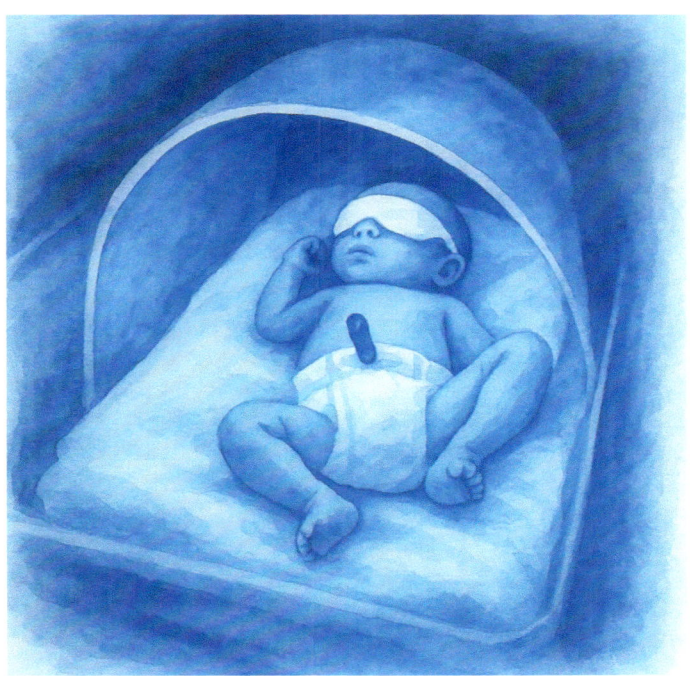

The moment of truth came with the next heel prick test. For Paul, the test showed that his bilirubin levels were high enough that he needed phototherapy, otherwise known as "going under the lights."

Phototherapy works by shining a special blue light over the baby's skin, which helps break down excess bilirubin so the liver can process it more easily. Paul had to spend several hours under the lights at a time, wearing a tiny eye mask to protect his eyes, while we kept a careful watch on him. Meanwhile Chris was just on the borderline of needing treatment, so he got to stay snuggled with us. Even then, we knew his turn might come if his levels crept up.

We were struggling with feeding because of what turned out to be severe tongue ties for both boys. A tongue tie is a tiny piece of tissue under the baby's tongue that stops them from moving it freely. It might seem minor, but it can turn breastfeeding into a bit of a wrestling match. Babies need to lift and extend their tongue to latch properly and move milk efficiently. With a tongue tie, they can't, which means they might suck ineffectively or chew at the nipple instead. Cue sore, cracked nipples, extra-long feeds, and the occasional frustrated "are we doing this right?" moment. If you suffer such difficulties urgently ask the question about getting checked for a tongue tie.

The consultant referred us to the infant feeding team. The specialist who looked after us was amazing. Paul was particularly poorly because of jaundice, and Chris was just on the edge of needing treatment. When the specialist first examined them, she helped Cath with positioning and latching to reduce pain. There was still a lot of pain, though, and the specialist quickly realised both boys had severe tongue ties, as bad as the photos in the information sheets. She arranged for them to be treated the very next day.

This made a huge difference. Although Paul still needed treatment for jaundice, the tongue tie correction helped them feed correctly and start to thrive.

By chance, the day she helped Cath, my sister was there meeting the twins for the first time, and as we all chatted with the feeding specialist, it turned out that she had lived just down the road from my sister. Then the conversation shifted to a PhD student researching some fascinating glass objects found in her back garden. I actually knew that student, as she'd come to look at some of our museum material. The feeding specialist then mentioned she was going to move, we discovered it was the same road as my parents. It's those little coincidences that make the world feel very small and make you wonder if you're in a museum-themed version of EastEnders.

Since then, we have bumped into the specialist a couple of times. Once when we gave her some eggs as a thank-you, and another time I spotted her with her daughter while driving past. I'm not sure if I called her a hero out loud when we said hi, but I definitely thought it. (Spoiler alert: she is a hero). Without her help and rapid intervention Cath definitely would not have been able to breastfeed the twins.

We were also lucky to be among the first group of multiple births in Southampton to have a special training session, the first since the Covid pandemic. That session helped us understand what to expect during delivery and afterwards. Part of the training mentioned jaundice and treatment, but it wasn't until later that we fully realised with multiples given they tend to be preterm jaundice treatment is pretty much guaranteed. This was one of the hardest times for us. The boys had been very close together in the womb, suddenly they were separated for treatment very soon after birth. That was difficult for them, and us.

With tongue ties and feeding difficulties, treating the twins was a real challenge. They didn't feed quickly, so we were told we needed a supplementary feed of 60–70 millilitres as well as breast feeding every three hours to flush out the jaundice. It was tough on their tiny tummies and emotionally draining. Their crying could probably have won awards. A terrible song stuck on repeat, and we were the only DJs who couldn't change the track.

Two things really helped us get through it. First, after the tongue-tie treatment, we discovered we could do the secondary top up feed with Paul without taking him out of his phototherapy cot. This meant he could stay under the light for an extra half hour after each breast feed, which made a big difference. Second, a consultant encouraged us to see the process as a team effort rather than a frustrating ordeal. She explained that every minute Paul wasn't under the light was a minute lost, time he'd have to catch up on later. If we wanted him to recover quickly and come home as soon as possible, we had to work together.

She challenged us to get each feed done in under 15 minutes: feeding, changing nappies, settling, putting the mask back on, then starting the next feed. We never quite hit 15 minutes, but we halved the time it took.

Cleaning up after a newborn who had started to poo was a particularly smelly, stressful challenge. At first, it was mostly meconium. This is a thick, sticky, dark green substance that's basically the baby's first poo, made up of everything he'd ingested in the womb. It's notoriously hard to clean, and trying to do it quickly while keeping Paul comfortable turned each nappy change into a race against both the clock and a very stubborn nappy.

By this point, Paul had been on and off the lights for three and a half days. Whenever it was time for a blood test, Cath would be with Chris looking through the window waiting for my expression and I'd help with the heel prick. Usually, people would wait for the midwife to come in and show them the graph, we both work with statistics and had spent far too long looking at graphs about bilirubin so right away I would know if it was good or bad. For days, it was bad, like black smoke in the Vatican, my expression said it all and Cath would know it was another 8 or 12 hours under the lights.

Finally, Paul's levels dropped significantly! We knew it was likely time to come off the lights and wait 12 hours to see if he was ready to go home. Those 12 hours were nerve-wracking. Earlier, his levels had been 200, if it was above 220 he would be back on the lights for the third time.

The tests came back and honestly I wanted to cry. 221… I was horrified, fearing another stint under the lights. Cath could tell right away looking across the corridor that I thought it was bad. By then, it was day 11 in the hospital, and we were exhausted. Thankfully, the midwife spoke with the consultant, who agreed we could go home. We had to return if Paul's condition worsened.

This all happened on the 19th of September. My 37th birthday, no less. By that point, I had been surviving mostly on M&S salads for too long. Cath's colleague had brought over a chili two days before, and our friend Nicky delivered a special meal the day after. Then mum and dad arrived on my birthday with incredible sandwiches from an award-winning butcher, a feast fit for royalty. The generosity of our friends, with meals that felt like tiny celebrations, made all the difference.

Even in our private room, we managed only an hour or two of sleep each night, thanks to tests, feeds, nappy changes, and the general discomfort of a sofa bed. But I can't complain, especially compared to other families who have had more difficult births where their partners could not stay.

Two moments from that time still stand out vividly. The first was Emma's face lighting up when she met the twins for the first time. She wore a T-shirt that said "Big Sister Emma," bought by one of her best friend's mums. They also had gifted matching newborn baby grows "Little Brother Chris" and "Little Brother Paul". Seeing her excitement and joy was unforgettable.

The second is the sound of the twins' cries for milk during those first 18 hours. They were more like little chirping birds "teehe he teehe he teehe…" one of the cutest, most helpless sounds imaginable. We even have a short video, which we occasionally watch. It still doesn't sound quite like babies, especially compared to the later lung-busting cries!

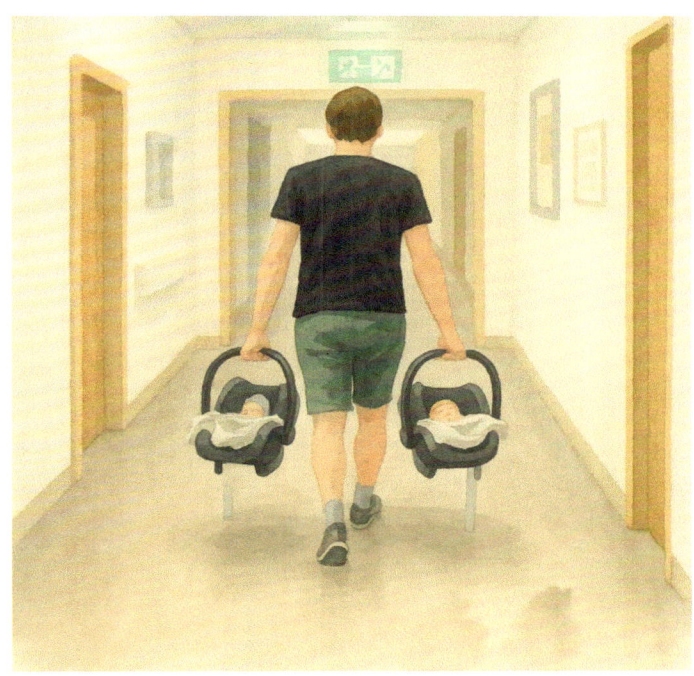

It was around 12.30 a.m. when we finally got home. Our cats, Timmy and Carter, rushed over, eager for attention, then quickly retreated upstairs to observe the boys from a safe distance. Clearly, they smelled… different. You could almost see their thought bubbles: "What on earth are these things? We never gave you permission to bring them inside. Kindly take them away. Thank you."

What We Wish We Had Known About Twin Births

The induction can be a marathon, not a sprint: We'd heard labour stories and Cath's active labour with Emma had been a three day slog. For us the drawn-out nature of induction, especially for twins, was something else entirely. Waiting around for staffing, shifts changing, and those vague "half an hour" estimates that stretch into hours felt like a lesson in patience we didn't quite sign up for. If someone had told us to pack snacks, comfy shoes, and a willingness to embrace 'hospital time' as its own strange universe, we'd have been better prepared.

Sudden theatre trips are very much a possibility: We thought we'd be in a nice, calm birthing room. Instead, once Dave-Dave did his acrobatics and flipped breech, everything shifted into a whirlwind. It was reassuring to have been prepped for the possibility of theatre. The speed of it still caught us off guard. Having a heads-up about how quickly things can escalate would have helped reduce the shock when the room suddenly filled with consultants, midwives, and all the paraphernalia.

Naming embryos isn't just a quirky idea, it's a survival mechanism: Naming them Dave and Dave-Dave made us smile through some pretty intense moments. It was a fun distraction and a way to personalise the chaos. We never expected to hear midwives cheering on Dave-Dave during labour, but it helped make the experience feel more manageable and a little less clinical.

Feeding multiples is a whole different challenge: Tongue ties, jaundice, and the slow, painful process of feeding and refeeding were emotionally exhausting. We wish we'd known just how much support and specialist help would make a difference.

Our feeding consultant became our hero, offering simple tips that made latching on much less challenging. It really can be tricky with twins. After a few months, we transitioned to a bottle around 7pm, which reduced some pressure for Cath.

Jaundice and treatment are almost guaranteed with twins, and the separation can be heartbreaking: We underestimated the emotional toll of seeing the boys apart, under different treatments, and having to 'force feed' them to clear jaundice and comforting their distress at being separated. Knowing this might happen, and that the hospital staff would work with us as a team, would have helped set realistic expectations.

Be prepared for a long stay: One thing we really wish we'd known from the start is just how long everything could take. We went in thinking induction would be a quick process, maybe a day or two at most, and that we'd be home celebrating with two new babies shortly after. Nope. It turned into an epic stay. Honestly, it felt like time slowed down to a crawl in that hospital.

Sandwiches for 10 days is dire, and friends' kindness means the world: After days of eating sandwiches, salads and hospital meals, the arrival of homemade chicken stew, chilis, award-winning sandwiches, and thoughtful meals from friends felt like little gifts of love that kept us going.

Finally, expect exhaustion and very limited sleep: Even when we were moved to a private room, rest was rare during the induction and post-birth. If someone had warned us that sleep deprivation would hit like a freight train and that surviving on snippets of sleep was the new normal, we might have stocked up on coffee and accepted the inevitability a little faster.

Bringing them home: the first days and weeks

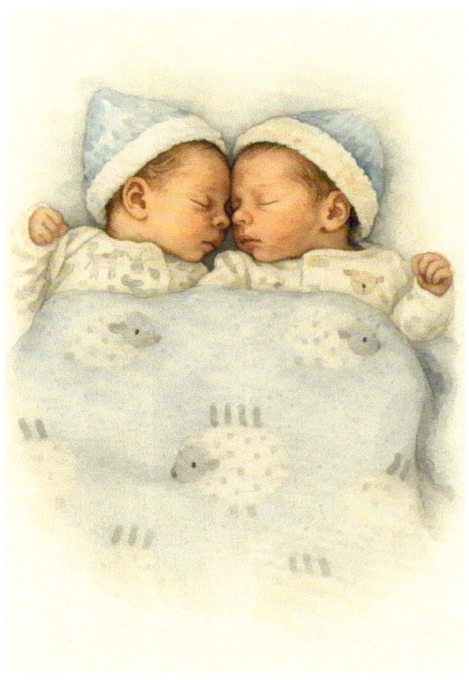

Looking back, there are only a handful of things we vividly remember from those early months. The rest is a bit of a blur due to severe sleep deprivation, endless battles with feeding and reflux, and more nappy changes than we thought physically possible. Life became an endless cycle of keeping two tiny humans alive and vaguely content. With twins, you quickly learn that organisation isn't optional. Getting them to sleep, poo, and eat roughly in sync is the only way you stand a chance of grabbing a breather yourself. When it worked, it felt like a small victory; when it didn't, chaos reigned.

Because of the sheer number of nappies we went through, one thing we decided very early on was that reusable nappies stashed in the attic were a non-starter. While we regularly feel a pang of environmental guilt, the idea of washing what comes out of them, especially during weaning and teething, was a bridge too far. On what for us was just a normal day with two, Emma suggested she should pay us £1 for every nappy she didn't have to change. Sadly, when she saw the day's total, she quickly withdrew the offer. We would have been £19 richer.

The first few months were really difficult because of the reflux. Both boys struggled with it, and it was heartbreaking. Even if we held them upright for 30 minutes after every feed, trying desperately to help the milk stay down, it would still come back up. You get used to a certain level of laundry with newborns, but this was Olympic-level.

Reflux is pretty common in babies, but it's especially common in premature ones. Their digestive systems just aren't fully developed yet. The main issue is the lower oesophageal sphincter. This is the little "valve" between the oesophagus and the stomach that's supposed to keep food and stomach acid where it belongs. In premature babies, it doesn't quite close properly, so instead of staying put, the milk makes a return journey, often mixed with stomach acid. Cue unsettled babies, endless outfit changes for everyone, and parents running on fumes.

It took an emotional toll too, especially on Cath, who would spend hours in the middle of the night feeding, holding, winding, and soothing only for it all to end in another round of sick and the cycle had to start all over again. The boys were already tiny, sitting way down on the growth charts at around the 7th and 9th centiles, and every lost feed felt like a setback. Weight gain was painfully slow. It made every ounce hard won and every weigh-in nerve-racking. Now, looking back, the change is staggering as by eleven months Paul was up on the 90th centile, a transformation that still amazes us. We attribute this to Italy leading to his love of homemade pizza.

Eventually, the GP prescribed Infant Gaviscon. It works by thickening the milk so it's less likely to come back up, which sounds brilliant in theory. At first, it did seem to help with the vomiting. But the supposed miracle cure had its dark side. A common side effect of Gaviscon causes constipation. For Chris, it was especially brutal. Suddenly we were faced with a miserable dilemma. Do we choose reflux and vomiting, or excruciating pain from constipation? After watching Chris scream in agony at night *for hours*, completely inconsolable we decided the Gaviscon just wasn't worth it.

So we went back to basics. Sometimes little changes helped. We raised the boys' bassinets with little wedges. The boys weren't lying flat, but they weren't sitting up either. This gentle slope helped gravity keep things heading the right way. It doesn't sound like much, but that little bit of tilt sometimes meant they'd sleep for an extra hour. And when you're living in the newborn trenches, an extra hour of sleep is worth its weight in gold.

As if reflux wasn't enough, from six weeks the boys had another party trick, one that terrifies people when they first see it. When they cried too hard, both Paul and Chris would simply stop breathing, turn blue, and pass out. We'd seen toddlers do the breath-holding thing mid-tantrum before, a short-lived protest that ends with a dramatic gasp. This seemed different, it could happen halfway through a feed, or mid-grizzle, with no warning. The first time it occurred, we went straight to the doctor. They were surprised, too, and sought specialist advice referred us on, only for the paediatrician to wave it off as if it were an everyday hiccup.

The NHS guidance might say this sort of thing can happen, but nothing prepares you for holding a baby who has suddenly gone floppy and blue. Most episodes last only 30 seconds, but when it is bad they can be passed out for around two minutes.

Two. Minutes!

Those are the longest 120 seconds of our lives. The textbooks and websites tend to be oddly blasé about it, as if you'll take it in your stride. When you've got *two* children capable of passing out at the same time, it's not something you shrug off. Luckily, when it first happened, both of us were there, so one could deal with each baby if needed.

We learned that the quickest fix was to blow gently on their faces, which usually forced them to take a breath. It became so routine for us that we'd warn anyone looking after them: "They might go blue, but just blow on their face and it might help." People would nod politely, clearly thinking we were exaggerating. Then it happened.

In Italy, for example, family friends were visiting for a couple of days. We gave them the usual warning, they smiled and waved it off. T hen both boys did it within minutes of each other. I think the realisation hit them hard: when we say it can get bad quickly, we're not joking. At a work BBQ, Cath's boss experienced a pretty bad episode. Something that a paediatrician dismissed as normal terrifies anyone who is unprepared, it is easy to see why.

Reflecting on the first few months, one thing that became a constant in our lives was how people looked at us with surprise because of how we handled the babies. It's nothing dangerous, but when you've got two babies to pick up, it is impossible to pick up both babies at the same time with two hands like you would a singleton unless you have grown extra arms. Instead, you find a safe way to scoop while making sure the other doesn't roll off a blanket, and it looks far more dramatic than it actually is. To us it's just practical, to others it is an entirely alien approach they would never contemplate with one. They watch us like we're auditioning for a circus act.

What makes it even funnier (and slightly maddening) is how many unsolicited opinions you get, often from people you've never met. Giving us tips on how we could use both hands (we still have not grown four arms). Imagine the challenges with triplets. We've had retired midwives on Southampton Common chastise us for not having the boys checked for jaundice when we obviously had, multiple times. We've had well-meaning strangers give us tips that "worked with their one baby" years before I was even born, while both our boys were screaming in stereo while I weave in between the oak trees, as if the logistics of twins are exactly the same. Spoiler: they're not.

The thing is, with one baby, you usually get two hands, one lap, and more time to do things slowly. With twins, you just don't have that luxury. Life with two is different, not unsafe, not careless, just… adapted. You learn to trust your judgement and find the path that works for your family. That doesn't mean ignoring advice, but it does mean filtering out the noise. Because if we've learned anything, it's that comparison really is the thief of joy. What worked for someone else and their single baby in 1968 when they just left them at the bottom of the garden to cry is not something we will ever try. And that's fine.

I said there are a few things I vividly remember from those first few months while the rest is a blur. Foolishly, I assumed the boys would love bath time. Nope. They absolutely hated it. For the first few minutes, they'd just sit there and scream their little heads off like extras in a very low budget horror movie (Scream 6: The *Bath*) while you tried to wash them. Imagine being a tiny human who has no idea why they're suddenly soaking wet, it's pretty confusing and scary! Paul in particular was the biggest bath-time grump. It took him ages to warm up to the idea that being in a tub could actually be fun.

Now, of course, they really enjoy it. I guess the difference is they can finally engage with the whole splashing and playing, making it fun instead of terrifying. An experienced twin parent shared the tip of two washing baskets in the bath rub so they could bath together but safely which the boys loved. Our new challenge is trying to stop two adventurous boys trying to crawl up the sloped end like going up a slide the wrong way before sliding back with a splash. Now they often cry because of the shock of the unexpected dunking when your sibling plays twin pin bowling.

Halloween was another early memory that sticks out. I seized the chance to dress the twins up. One of the fun things about having twins is that you can go for either cute or amusing. That year, I dressed them as Jack Skellington. It was the only outfit I could really find that I thought would work as they were still in tiny baby clothes (less than 5lb).

In future years, I have plenty of other ideas. For example, I want to use our garden trolley to create a miniature Jurassic Park, with the twins in dinosaur outfits and me wearing a hat to complete the scene. Sadly, they're not girls, so I couldn't dress them as the creepy twins from *The Shining*, but the possibilities for my own amusement really are endless.

For reasons only children seem to fully understand, a lot of kids find nappy changes absolutely fascinating. They'll stand there, wide-eyed, like they're watching a nature documentary in real life. Sometimes they're transfixed by the sheer mechanics of it all. The poo, the wipes, creams, fastenings, a baby wriggling like an eel on the mat. Sometimes it's just the novelty of seeing something they know is usually hidden.

One boy had been watching us for a good five minutes, completely engrossed, before he suddenly broke his silence joking "His willy is bigger than mine!". It was the kind of entirely inappropriate comment only a child could get away with, and it stopped us in our tracks. We just had to laugh.

Emotional Realities

Bonding with twins is a joy… once you've survived the chaos. You get to see their tiny personalities emerge almost immediately: one wriggles more, one murmurs in a higher pitch, one after a few failed attempts likes the bath while the other screams bloody murder. Every feed, nappy, and cuddle is a double adventure, and double the mess.

Parenting multiples comes with its own unique emotional load. Guilt and self-doubt are frequent visitors, particularly if one twin fusses more than the other. Comparing babies with their peers becomes inevitable, and parents have to remind themselves constantly that each baby develops at their own pace. Anxiety about growth, development, and health is common, particularly if either baby was premature or needed extra care.

You will also at times compare both of your children with each other, it is sometimes useful and sometimes isn't. Ours are fascinatingly different given they were genetically identical at conception. Comparison did allow us at least to spot some medical issues such as torticollis and hearing problems caused by glue ear.

Support is crucial. For you that may be family, friends, and health professionals or online groups such as a local Facebook group for multiples. Sharing experiences, both triumphs and disasters, helps normalise the chaos and provides reassurance that yes, other parents have survived this too.

The help of friends and family in those early weeks was a god send, especially a food train set up for us by Jude so we had an evening meal sorted at the very least for the first three weeks. Lunches for a while were sorted as we had been given some batch cooked meals by Regan and Alex.

Practical Tips for the Early Weeks

Meal prep and support: Have easy meals ready, and accept help without guilt. If someone offers a lasagne or a fish pie, take it.

Tag-team sleep: Rotate spells during the night with your partner or support person to get longer stretches. Otherwise have a system where one person does the morning shift so you can nap. Even two hours can revitalise you. Some people myself included are surprisingly difficult to stir when so fast asleep and get grumpy if they do, Cath deserves a medal for taking this grumpiness so well most of the time.

Feeding strategies: Tandem feeding or synchronised bottle feeds can save your sanity.

Prepare for mess: Multiple babies equals multiple nappy poopocalypses, vomit incidents, and laundry piles. Accept it.

Take mental health seriously: Postpartum anxiety and depression for both parents is real. Early support matters.

Double (or triple) kit up: You may have thought you were prepared but we needed more spare muslins, spare outfits (for babies and you), and more nappies. Honestly, more than you think you'll ever need.

Say yes to visitors only when it works for you: Take time to settle in, you have two! Also if friends want to see the babies, ask them to bring milk, fold laundry, or hold a baby so you can shower.

Lower the bar: Forget spotless kitchens and matching outfits. Surviving counts as winning in the early weeks.

Sleeping in stereo: nights, naps, and finding rhythms

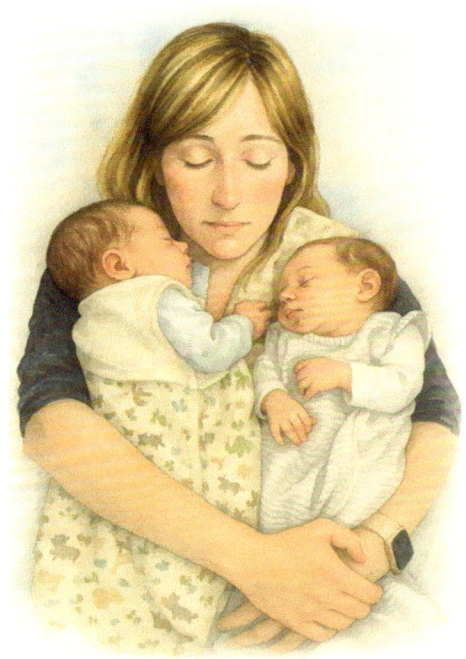

Sleep with twins is… complicated. From the start, our nights were punctuated by regular wake-ups for feeding, nappy changes, and the kind of tummy troubles that test every ounce of patience you didn't know you had. Reflux, colic, and mysterious aches meant they rarely slept for more than an hour or two at a stretch. They were almost never in sync. Even now at a year, Chris still often wakes every hour, while Paul can *sometimes* stretch it to a slightly more civil five hours.

Late-night full-feed vomiting due to reflux was soul-destroying, and every so often we were treated to the classic "exploding nappy." To add to the ambiance, we experimented with alternatives to white noise. For example, the Bridgerton soundtrack, in the hope that harps and flutes might somehow calm them. The results were... mixed.

There's something deeply peaceful about watching them sleep. Finally quiet, finally still. Sometimes they end up curled in the strangest positions, bums stuck up in the air like little baby hedgehogs attempting a handstand.

When both twins wake simultaneously, it can feel like a full-blown emergency. Our survival strategies included:

Divide and conquer: Cath would feed, I would hold them upright or change them, or vice versa.

Batch prep: Keeping bottles and nappies ready in every room saved precious minutes.

Deep breathing: It doesn't make them sleep, but it keeps your nerves intact.

Even with these strategies, some nights were disasters. I vividly remember one evening when the boys were two months oldwhen I persuaded Cath to go to see They Might Be Giants which we had book two years earlier. I barely survived 7pm–11pm because we had run out of expressed milk after the reflux struck. More recently, both were utterly apoplectic when Cath and Emma went to see her cousin Tom perform in his school production of *Matilda*. The sadness, frustration, and sheer tiredness in these moments are real, for us and for them.

We tried to wake them, feed them, and change them at the same time to create a rhythm. Some days, it worked beautifully.

Other days, it was a futile attempt to synchronise two tiny, unpredictable people. Moses baskets didn't suit them, and getting them to nap at home was usually unsuccessful. The buggy became the default nap spot. A flexible routine, rather than a rigid schedule, became our saving grace.

Safety was always a priority. Sudden infant death syndrome (SIDS), falls, and nodding off on the sofa are real risks. Even when exhaustion tempted us to "just lie down for a minute," we reminded ourselves that a few extra minutes of vigilance is better than an accident.

We learned a few things along the way:

Next-to-me sleepers were lifesavers for fleeting night feeds.

Swaddling and sleep sacks helped with reflux and restlessness.

Rocking twins gets harder fast, rocking an 11kg baby to sleep is a very different workout than rocking a 2kg one.

Flexible expectations: Sometimes the best you can do is for everyone to have a 20-minute nap.

Some parents swear their babies sleep like angels in the car, and even manage that magical transfer from car seat to cot just before bedtime. For us, that's not just rare, it's practically a myth.

Most of the time, we get the twin apocalypse. The boys don't just cry. They scream. Take the drive to Bluestone, for example. From Cardiff to the resort, roughly two hours in the car, they screamed.

Both of them. *The entire way.*

And not just any crying, but that relentless breathe–scream–breathe–scream routine that makes you question every decision you've ever made in life.

We tried everything: stopping, feeding, soothing, swapping toys, desperate singing. This was usually by Emma long suffering and trapped in the back, gamely trying to keep them calm while slowly losing the will to live. In the end, we bought her headphones so she could zone out and do other things if we have a hellish journey. It's honestly one of the best investments we've ever made.

The car woes were not just Wales. When we drove to Kent to pick up a Burley bike trailer and stopped to see my cousin Maria, the journey home from near Leatherhead was… well, let's just say it aged us all a decade. On our whistle-stop tour of the north, the stretch from Wolverhampton down was just as bad. The main conclusion? Car naps don't work for us. Not at bedtime. Not for naps. Not even for five minutes. Unless, of course, we want them to bloody stay awake. Then, and only then, they drift off like little angels.

These days as they are a bit older our routines have evolved, now we have dinner, bath time, milk and stories. We've settled into a few well-loved daily rituals which include a handful of books that the boys absolutely adore. *Zog* is always a hit, and recently they've been getting into *Room on the Broom* as well as *The Gruffalo* (we now have a copy with a puppet) all by Julia Donaldson. But their favourite, the one they return to again and again, is *Owl Babies*.

For those unfamiliar with it, *Owl Babies* is about how three owlets react when they think their mother has gone, only to discover she's just popped out hunting. Sorry for ruining the detailed plot...

Of course, we've given it a very personal twist: whenever the baby owls call out lines like "I want my mummy," in our household, they are Emma, Paul, and Chris. You can probably guess why.

Reading it together has become a performance in itself. Often, I narrate while one of the boys tries to eat the corner of the page. We've read it so many times now that we know exactly which lines are coming next, so Cath often chimes in with the best mummy owl voice: "What's all the fuss? You knew I'd come back!"

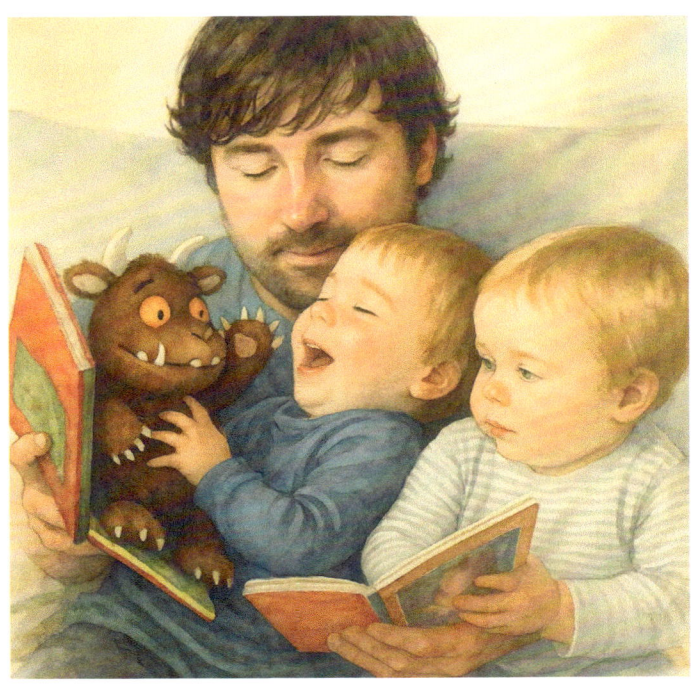

We've moved from a single cot to two conjoined Montessori floor beds as they were best for us in the space we have available. Sleep though has never been a strong point of the boys and they struggle to make it through a full sleep cycle.

Chris, who even now seems to think sleep should come in one-hour intervals, outdid himself one particularly memorable night during the heatwave. We could hear crying on the monitor, so we went upstairs to settle them. Often, if we catch them at that early stage, all that is needed is a gentle "shhhhh" and a bum pat. But this time was different. I found him standing on his Montessori floor bed, tiny hands gripping the top edge, screaming directly into the fan like a baby Michael Jackson rehearsing *Earth Song*. The sheer drama of it, the hair blowing back, the anguished wail. He had a reluctant audience in us as well as the wind machine, and all he needed was a backing track (or his brother to add harmonics).

Reflections

While their cries and tears have grown louder, in some ways it's easier now. We can usually work out what's wrong more quickly, rather than cycling through a checklist of milk? poo? vomit? Tummy spasm. Sleep with twins is a blend of improvisation, patience, and tiny victories. There are triumphs, be it a long nap in sync or a five-hour stretch at night, and there are disasters. The benefit of us getting so little sleep is we have very little memory of the more challenging moments. Sharing our honest experiences, from double wake-ups to routines that worked (and spectacularly failed), is our way of saying: you are not alone, and it is possible to survive this stage, even if your own sleep is mostly a distant memory.

The nap wars

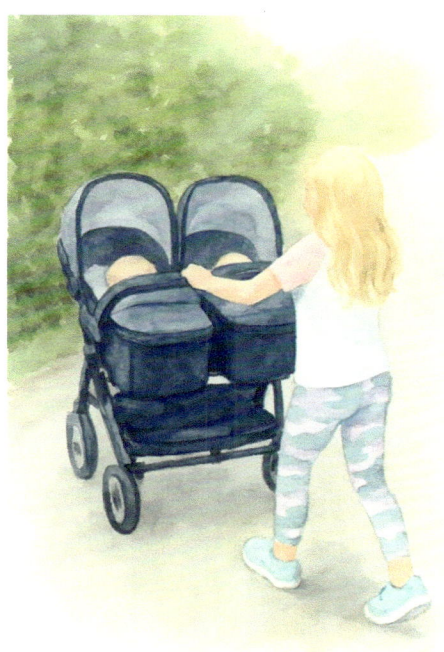

Naps, when the boys were really, really young, could happen anywhere. Sometimes they fell asleep on a shoulder. When they were tiny, you could literally hold them in one hand and they'd snooze like little kittens. Other times we put them in the bassinet and took them out for a little walk. They just slept wherever they pleased, if they slept at all!

Their day now starts at seven regardless of the previous nights challenges. Breakfast is the first order of business. These days it's proper food rather than milk. Porridge with some fruit or Weetabix though it's always an experiment. You quickly learn that babies don't always show their hand the first time they try something. Kiwi, for example, was met with blank refusal for weeks, but with teeth now in play it's a completely different game. If you have not prepared enough they will certainly let you know.

The first nap usually falls between 8.30 and 9.00, ideally for about an hour. The only reliable way to get them down has been the buggy. The cot at home has never been a success and the car is *very* hit and miss. But there's a fine line. If they sleep too long, it throws out the entire day. In fact, it's often worse than them sleeping too little. More than once Cath had to remind me, and the grandparents, that letting them snooze for two and a half hours in the morning was not actually a victory.

By 10.30 they're awake, ready for play, a little feed, and then some lunch. Their main nap of the day comes at around 1.00, again usually on foot. This is the big one, if we miss the window, the late afternoon "witching hour" is guaranteed to be unbearable. We used to offer a third, late-afternoon nap, but that's long gone, like nights where we got to actually sleep. I've also been trying to figure out what kind of witchcraft nursery uses to get fifteen to twenty babies to sleep all at once. Their answer? "They're just very tired." Sure, but I like to imagine it's a bit more mystical than that.

Even with the best-laid plans, naps can fall apart for any number of reasons. When they were younger, a particularly sad moment for one baby, often reflux-induced, could wake the other, creating what we fondly called a "cacophony of sadness." There's also the ever-present risk of a big poo. I don't need to explain why that makes sleep difficult.

Other threats lurk everywhere. Stopping mid-walk, people wanting to say hello without permission or lifting up the buggy hood. All these interruptions can derail a nap. You also get the very sympathetic looks from passersby when two absolutely apoplectic twins are refusing to go down for their morning or afternoon nap. I've discovered my headphones' noise-cancelling element is surprisingly useful, but mostly you just have to persist. Amble on, over rough ground or gravel, and hope that something, suddenly, clicks and allows them to settle. A gentle bit of weaving. It's difficult for people to predict where I'm going because we're pushing what feels like a tank.

Sometimes the risk of waking extends to excursions like the supermarket. You quickly get used to rocking the buggy backwards and forwards to keep the boys asleep while trying to navigate a trolley. One thing I will genuinely miss about those short, chaotic trips to the shops is the sheer spectacle of it all when you take them both by yourself. One twin asleep in the buggy the other in a trolley wide-eyed and thrilled at the world, while I try not to cause absolute chaos for everybody else in the supermarket. We have also braved these excursions when both boys are awake. The boys get very excited about what's in the trolley: you'll see Paul trying to break into a packet of plums while Chris is gnawing on a packet of Jammy Dodgers that are definitely not for him, although he very much wishes they were. They absolutely loved it. Sadly, now that we're mostly doing online shopping, this little adventure will be a thing of the past, though it will probably help our bank balance.

There are days that you just have to give up on routine and go with the flow. One day during Daddy Daycare the twins going blue derailed the nap plan, I went to work to see my colleague Jess. She absolutely loves the twins and getting their regular "twupdates." On a Monday, we decided to sit outside her office where there is a disabled access ramp. The boys rampaged along it for ages. The ramp is probably six metres long, slightly precarious, and a tiny bit dangerous. No wonder they adored it. They raced up and down as fast as they could, giggling away, before pausing, sometimes for a little snack, or in Chris's case, lying face down as if he was about to fall asleep right on the ramp itself. Occasionally they got a little bit too close to the edge, which terrified Jess a little.

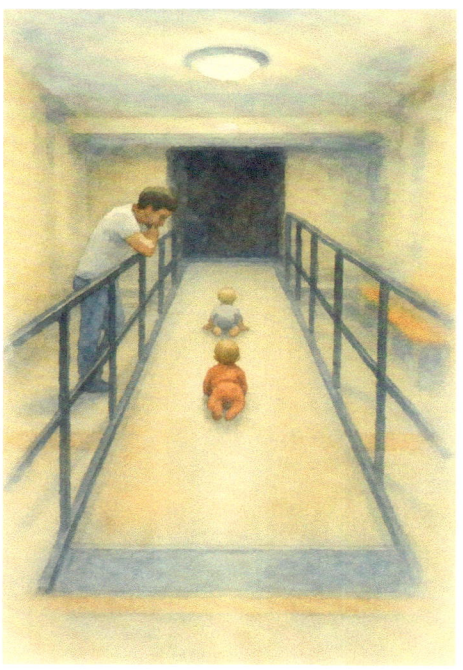

The ramp actually worked really well. After an hour of racing up and down it, the boys were completely exhausted, and on the way back they fell asleep in the buggy. In the future, I might look for something with handrails to stop the twins from trying to dive off headfirst, helping to alleviate any stress others might experience. A good tip for anyone struggling with naptime is to find a safe way to let them burn off all their energy first, ramps are optional extras.

One thing we've never had any success with is self-soothing. I can see how it would make life a lot easier if the boys could learn to settle themselves back to sleep, even just after a little cough, but for us it's been impossible. The main challenge is that they can go blue and pass out if left alone whenever they are distressed so we have to keep a very close eye on them day and night. The other issue is that if one wakes up crying for long enough, it often wakes the other, too.

Self-soothing is one of those mystical elements people tell you works, but for us, it simply never has. I'd love to share the secret to getting twins to self-soothe, but truthfully, I'm still holding out for someone to show *me* the magic trick. Preferably one that doesn't involve oxygen deprivation and passing out (and turning them blue in the process).

From eleven months we started teetering on the edge of losing the morning nap altogether. This is both liberating and miserable. Paul, especially, lets us know his feelings about tiredness, today's protest involved trying to dive headfirst out of his highchair rather than accept kiwi fruit. Grandparents struggle even more to get them down for the morning nap, sometimes managing only thirty minutes, which just confirms we're right on the cusp of losing it. I suspect nursery will finish the job.

They start nursery at the ripe old age of 361 days, just shy of their first birthday, and nursery runs on an entirely different timetable, lunch at eleven, naps earlier, and a more structured routine. I wouldn't be surprised if the morning nap vanishes overnight.

Of course, it's not all battles and chaos. There are some unexpected benefits to this nap-driven life. Between the morning and lunchtime naps, I regularly cover ten to fifteen miles a day on foot so that Cath can rest. Back when there was a third nap, it was even more. All that wandering, whether around the Common or down to Riverside Park in Bitterne, has meant I've lost a stone and worn out a couple of pairs of shoes.

The changing seasons are especially interesting to the boys now. When they wake up, if I'm still around the Common, they just stare at things with wonder. In August, the heat wave meant trees started losing leaves much earlier than usual, sometimes falling on their heads. Moments like these remind you that what we might see as mundane such as the changing of the seasons, are really quite special. You notice the little things in a way you wouldn't if you were behind a desk all day.

In other chapters, we've tried to offer hints, tips, and little lessons learned from our mistakes or things that have worked. As you can see, we really don't have any surefire answers. If there is a magic formula for getting twins to nap peacefully and self-soothe without turning blue, we'd very much like to know it ourselves.

Feeding the crowd: breast, bottle, and beyond

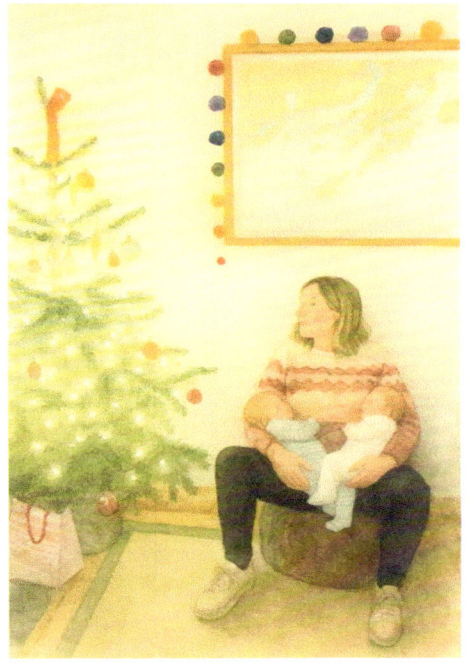

I breastfed, which was wonderful but not without its challenges. Early on, I felt there was extra pressure to make sure the boys drank enough to help flush out jaundice, adding another layer of stress to every feed. A piglet-feeding pillow made tandem feeds more manageable, though reflux sometimes reminded us that comfort is relative. Expressing milk was another adventure where 5am pumping sessions make me sympathise with dairy cows. A dear friend even sent me their pumping playlist and top tips for getting in the mood in the early hours of the morning.

The hospital feeding consultant was a lifesaver. They had a nipple measuring tool which meant women could have comfortable well-fitting pumping flanges. Most womens nipples are around 15-17mm wide whereas the standard flange that comes with pumps is 24mm as it was based on a prototype made by a daily farmer based on udders.

Little tweaks in positioning yourself and the babies can make a massive difference to my comfort as well as feeding efficiency. Their simple, practical tips made latching on much less tricky. I had also never heard of breast compressions when Emma was young and it definitely helped up the boys intake in the early days.

There are times that we have to resort to tandem feeding. When out and about the boys are easily distracted which can be stressful. We'll never forget a day trip to Burley, in the New Forest, where both were suddenly mesmerised by well, anything. It included passing dogs, leaves, and birds resulting in a lot of sympathetic looks from passersby. A large lightweight scarf became our secret weapon, offering modesty, a little warmth, and a barrier against inevitable milk dribbles.

Sometimes late-night feeds ended with unexpected explosions: reflux turning into vomit, or one of the boys spraying milk from the bottle in a perfectly straight arc. There were moments when we sat there, drenched, burping one baby while trying not to slip on the other's dribble, wondering if anyone else survived twin nights like this. It was soul-destroying at the time, but now it's one of those stories that makes us laugh, mostly because we lived to tell the tale.

Supplementing with bottles brought its own lessons, including mastering the awkward art of holding one baby while keeping the other content. Cluster feeds, those marathon sessions, tested patience, endurance, and sometimes your very understanding of time. After a few months, we transitioned to a bottle around 7 pm, which eased some pressure for Cath and gave us a bit more flexibility in the evening.

We spent ages experimenting with the best way to feed two babies from bottles. Feeding two at the same time can feel like a logistical exercise that should come with a flowchart. Chris had a particularly sensitive stomach, so on the advice of a consultant we went with a formula that was supposed to be gentler on him. Our health visitor reminded us that all the first milk infant formulas are nutritionally the same regardless of their pricing and marketing. Once you commit to a brand, though, you quickly discover that swapping can cause chaos. Babies don't always take kindly to a sudden change in taste or texture. Whether that's universal or just our two being fussy is hard to say, but we weren't brave enough to push our luck too much.

Of course, like everything baby-related, everyone has an opinion on how you should feed them. People who haven't been up at 3 a.m. with two screaming infants will happily tell you what "worked for their single baby" or why formula is either a godsend or awful. The truth is, you just find the balance that works for your family and block out the noise.

In practice, we ended up settling into a routine: mostly breastfeeding, with one bottle feed in preparation for bedtime and then a "dream feed." For anyone who hasn't come across the term before, a dream feed is when you slip a bottle into your sleeping baby's mouth late at night (usually around 10–11 p.m.)

in the hope that they'll take it without properly waking up, and then sleep for a longer stretch afterwards. It's a bit like topping up a petrol tank before a long drive, except the car sometimes burps, spits half of it back at you, and then still wakes up five minutes later anyway.

When they were smaller, bottle-feeding them in their bouncers worked surprisingly well. They'd happily kick away, bouncing themselves gently while gripping the bottoms of their bottles, and for a brief glorious spell it felt like we'd cracked the code. Of course, it didn't last. The moment they got strong enough to bounce more enthusiastically, bottles went flying and the whole thing descended into chaos. At least they learnt about gravity.

Nowadays, their preferred method is a little more unconventional - standing up, lor eaning against the sofa, while you awkwardly hold the bottle at the right angle. Sitting down and feeding them like you would a "normal" baby just doesn't cut it anymore. It might look odd to anyone watching, but like so much else with twins, you quickly learn that whatever works is the right way.

Through it all, we learned that what worked one day might fail spectacularly the next. Some positions, pillows, or timings would be magic one afternoon and useless the next. But every small victory, be it that both babies latched at the same time, or finally stayed focused for a five-minute feed really felt monumental. Spills, burps, random dribbles, and sympathetic stares became part of the story, reminders that twin feeding is messy, unpredictable, and, in its own chaotic way, memorable.

Weaning times two: first foods and feeding fails

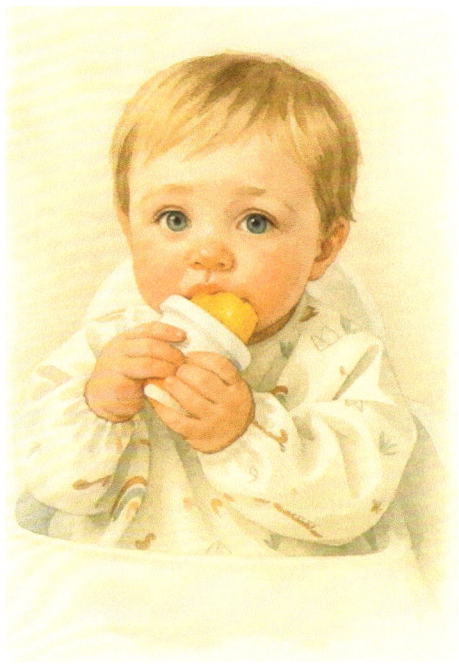

Emma and I had this grand plan for the boys' six-month birthday: their very first taste of proper food. After much discussion (and Emma's conviction that it was the perfect starter), we settled on avocado. Interesting taste, unusual texture, and apparently very on-trend if you believe parenting blogs. But the night before, Cath gave them broccoli. Yes, broccoli. This act of culinary sabotage is now firmly enshrined in family history, and Cath will never live it down.

The avocado reveal itself was… underwhelming. We expected squeals of delight or at least a curious gum. Instead, we got two tiny faces radiating pure suspicion, as if we'd offered them a plate of homework. The books will tell you, "Don't give up, babies may need to try a food 20 or more times before accepting it." 20 times! After the expressions we got, eight more attempts with avocado sounded like a cruel and unusual punishment. These days though they love it in an avocado and cream cheese wrap.

Of course, we still experimented. Sweet potato was an instant hit, prunes unexpectedly won applause, and Chris revealed a true love of strawberries. We even made it competitive by offering two foods side by side to see which Chris picked first. This turned into a long-running joke until Italy, four months later, when a fresh, sun-ripened melon finally toppled the British strawberry from its throne. Parenting tip: sometimes the best weaning strategy is a plane ticket.

One thing we've often discovered when introducing new things to the boys is that they tend to assume anything small and red must be a strawberry. For example, Chris would often be very unhappy that we had not given him peppers stuffed with cheese. In his mind, they were strawberries and we had committed treason. We've had similar issues with radishes and cherry tomatoes although now that they have so many teeth, that's probably less of a problem.

Then there are snacks. When we were at Lulworth Cove, it was the first time we decided to let them try an ice lolly. We bought a Jude's mini milk to share between the boys. Paul clearly thought it was going to be yoghurt, and his face said it all.

We think he experienced brain freeze for the first time, he tried to eat a good chunk all at once! But after that initial shock, he realised he actually liked it. His expression slowly changed from revulsion, to confusion, to delight, and then about 35 seconds later to absolute disappointment because the ice cream was gone. So now, anything that looks like a strawberry or ice cream is very, very popular with them. It has made sneaky stops for ice cream much harder.

The thing about weaning twins is that it isn't just about *what* they eat, but how much, how often, and the sheer scale of the mess. Two highchairs, two bibs, two sets of flailing arms and usually at least one child refusing what the other one loves. There were days it felt less like a family meal and more like running a canteen for very fussy (and very sticky) zoo animals. We quickly learned that wipes needed to be stationed in every room, the washing machine was never off, and that cooking in bulk was the only way to stay sane. Emotionally, it could be tough too. You'd spend ages steaming and mashing some lovingly prepared new food, only to have it flung across the room by both of them in unison. But the flip side was pure joy, watching them discover new tastes and textures, seeing their little faces light up with something they loved, and slowly realising that this was how they would grow strong.

What's been fascinating to watch is how quickly they've developed and how this has changed what they eat. Their teeth came through en masse, four at a time, so they had eight teeth (six at the top and two at the bottom) before they were even one, enabling them to move from gumming to tearing off chunks. That early dental head start meant they could tackle a surprising variety of foods, from crunchy breadsticks to bits of pasta. Alongside the teeth came dexterity, their little opposible fingers and thumbs suddenly working together so they could pick up even the tiniest morsels. With orzo, it often takes a few attempts, but they're stubbornly persistent. There's something oddly mesmerising about watching such small hands working with complete focus.

On the final day of editing this book, Cath had Paul on her lap while trying to eat. We did our best to keep him occupied with a breadstick snack, since the boys had already eaten dinner and were having their evening bottle. Paul, however, decided it was far more entertaining to dip his breadstick into Cath's pasta. He thought it was brilliant. Cath, on the other hand, was less than thrilled to discover soggy breadstick floating among her stuffed pasta. Perhaps it was his way of adding the final edit.

Looking back now, it's hard to believe both boys started life so small, both below the 10th centile when they were born. Through all the mess, the broccoli betrayal, and the endless battles with bibs, they've turned into brilliant eaters. Paul has climbed to the 90th centile, while Chris, our little fruit bat, would happily live on strawberries, melon, and grapes if we let him. These days, homemade pizza, orzo, and spaghetti are firm favourites, and mealtimes feel less like survival mode and more like a proper family ritual but with a lot of mess.

Weaning twins has been chaotic, hilarious, and downright exhausting. But it's also been one of the most rewarding parts of parenting so far. To see them grow from tiny, fragile babies into sturdy little boys who love their food feels like watching a miracle unfold every day. It's horrifically messy, noisy, and not at all how we imagined, but we wouldn't change it for the world.

Pouches: Helpful Tool or Slippery Slope?

Food pouches are one of those inventions that seem designed purely for the sanity of parents. You're in a café, one baby's wailing, the other is trying to eat the table leg, and a pouch of pureed pear can feel like a lifesaver. And they are, in moderation. The problem is that it's very easy to lean on them a bit too much. They're convenient, yes, but they also come at a price, literally, since buying a pouch is far more expensive than giving them an actual banana, and nutritionally too.

When fruit is blitzed and processed like that, the sugars behave differently in the body, and it's not quite the same as chomping on the real thing. So aside from prunes we used pouches sparingly: great for emergencies, a godsend for travel, but not the backbone of the boys' diet. Our rule of thumb was: if you can peel it and mash it with a fork in less than a minute, you don't need to buy it in a pouch.

We've chosen not to give the boys things like fruit and veggie melts or vegetable puffs that vanish the moment they hit their mouths. While some parents find them handy, to us they don't feel especially nourishing, a bit like filling up on cardboard. Instead, we try to offer real fruit and vegetables, so the boys get to explore proper tastes and textures while also building good eating habits. If they need a simple snack, we always have breadsticks at the ready.

Managing the Mess, Routine, and Nutrition

The mess is relentless. We got into the habit of laying down old cardboard boxes under the highchairs, and we thought we owned more bibs than some people have socks (but then we had to buy even more). But beyond just cleaning, we found routine was the real sanity-saver. We tried to keep mealtimes fairly regular, not just for the boys' hunger cues but for our own sense of order. As for nutrition, variety was our main aim: lots of colours, lots of textures, and a balance between familiar "safe" foods and the occasional curveball. It didn't always work, but the exposure seemed to pay off. We learned that a rejected food wasn't wasted if you tried it again a week later, sometimes it came back into fashion like flared jeans.

What to Buy, What to Skip

There's an entire industry devoted to weaning gadgets, and we tried a fair few. Some were worth their weight in gold: suction bowls that actually stayed stuck (most don't), long-sleeved bibs that one day will double as art smocks, and a decent hand blender for quick purees. But a lot of things were, frankly, useless. If you're weaning twins, space and sanity are at a premium, so our advice is simple: buy practical, skip the gimmicks, and remember that the best weaning tool you own is probably already in your kitchen drawer.

One of the best discoveries we made far too late was rolls of disposable paper tablecloths. They're brilliant for minimalising food waste when eating outside, but even better when you're in a pub or restaurant and don't want to leave the floor looking like a war zone. You just roll one out, tuck it under the highchairs, and it catches almost everything. Afterwards, you can gather it up, bin it, and walk away without cursing as you try to scrape baked-on pasta from someone else's carpet. Honestly, I wish we'd found them earlier, they would have saved hours of scrubbing and a fair amount of parental rage.

Tiny tornadoes: twins on the move

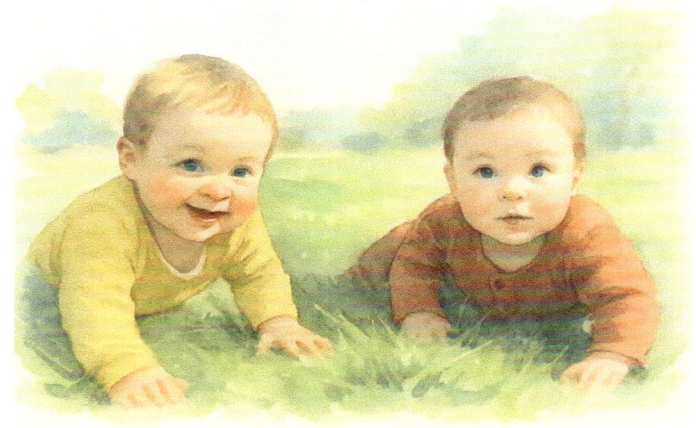

Our twins started crawling at around eight months and it's safe to say that from that day on, every day brings a certain amount of chaos. It was usually funny but not always easy to handle, especially if you're solo-parenting. Cath went back to work when the boys were eleven months. Therefore, most days either Cath's at work or I am, so one of us ends up looking after both boys alone. On weekends my mornings started with taking them for a walk, giving them breakfast, and getting them down for a nap so Cath can catch up on sleep. Then, for the rest of the morning and afternoon, Cath takes over and I tended to take them out for their afternoon nap.

Both boys are adventurous, but rarely in the same direction. The exception is when Paul makes a certain noise that causes Chris to immediately drop whatever he's doing and charge after him. Chris makes a similar noise from time to time, but Paul currently has glue ear in both ears and can't hear certain pitches. It's a small mercy in some ways, because otherwise the chaos would be doubled. Instead, Chris calls him, then looks over in confusion when Paul doesn't respond, only to see him still happily gnawing on whatever treasure he's found.

The twins remind Richard's parents Alison and Chris of him. For a while they used to call me "Busy Bum." You can probably guess why. I was always on the move, crawling, then running around just in a nappy. It's actually quite entertaining now, especially when you watch how a baby moves with a really full nappy, a bit like a goose. Watching a baby with a *really* full nappy does have its risks though. Fast forward a bit, and thanks to some former colleagues, I was handed a new nickname: "Thuglet."

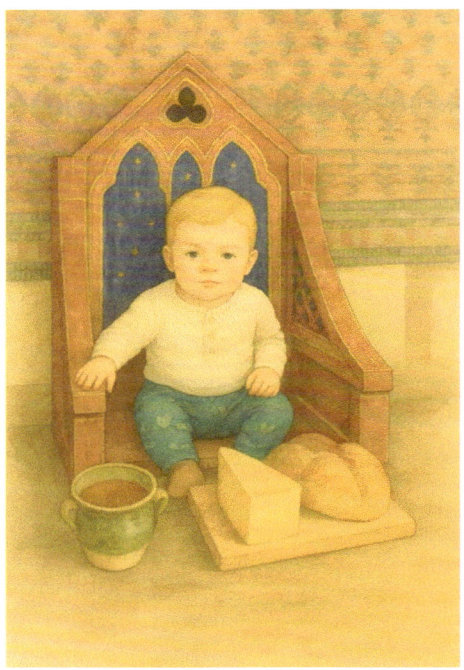

That nickname has now passed down to the next generation, only now there are two little thuglets. I took them to see Helen and Lily at the Medieval Merchant House in Southampton, and, true to form, they launched straight into a full thuglet rampage. It is a bit awkward when you are a curator and your son climbs onto a chair in the exhibition, sits there like he's the head of the medieval household, and then discovers the children's toys upstairs. Within minutes, there was a foam sword battle, one sword snapped and immediately became a snack, and then they were gnawing on the toy throwing axes and wearing the rope hoops as crowns. Thuglets gonna thuglet.

Watching them go about their daily business is a bit like watching badgers trying to break into a chicken coop. Badgers are small but incredibly determined and can cause quite a lot of chaos in a coop. These boys aren't out hunting chickens, but they have a singular mission, to get where they want to go, no matter what.

Instead of navigating around obstacles, they plough straight through them. Just like when you go on a Bear Hunt, Sometimes that even means barging straight through their brother, who's not always thrilled with this tactic. Like badgers, the boys are short, stocky, and incredibly strong. Honestly, they'd make perfect hookers on a rugby pitch. No one has invented infant rugby yet, which is probably for the best although there is rugby tots!

Although they're identical, you can usually tell them apart from their faces, it's just harder from above or behind. Their personalities, though, couldn't be more different.

We're really lucky to have two incredibly smiley children and that is why strangers are so engaged with them. Chris, in particular, will often smile back even through tears. The glint in his eye says "I'm about to cause trouble." And, to be fair, he usually is. He's the adventurous one, always finding a way to get up to mischief. If either of them is going to wander off or put themselves in a precarious spot such as on a bag of giant Jenga tower blocks eating a bit of orange, it's *always* Chris.

During labour, I thought he was spinning round because he didn't want to leave. Now I think he was just setting off on his first adventure. He's a bit of a lemming. Happy to crawl straight off a ledge, so you have to watch him closely. I've pulled off some impressive one-armed catches to stop disaster, the best being when he was about to launch himself off some decking. Another time when I held both boys he squirmed as I held him single handed and I had to grab him mid air. It was a catch a sportster would be proud of whereas Cath's face mostly said "were off to A&E".

Paul, on the other hand, is equally smiley but more measured. Unless food is involved, in which case he dives in head-first. He tends to think before he acts. He'll study something from every angle and touching it with his Peter Pointer finger before deciding what to do. By this time Chris is already halfway through doing it. Give Paul a new toy and he'll poke, prod, and turn it over in his hands; Chris will have already worked out how to dismantle it and is trying to post the pieces through the cat flap.

Childproofing for Two

Childproofing for one baby is fiddly, childproofing for two can felt like a very budget version of a house redesign. The boys see safety gates as climbing frames and anything closed as a personal challenge. Generally something closed draws much more attention. If one doesn't figure it out, the other usually will, it's a sort of tag-team mischief. On a good day, you get about 24 hours of peace before they've worked out a way around whatever you've put in place.

Certain spots in the house are repeat offenders. The corner of the kitchen where the cat food lives is a favourite. It is apparently a ready-made snack station for a hungry twin on the move. The fridge is another go to for the twins especially if we leave milk on the lowest shelf in the door. Emptying the dishwasher is now a race against time before one of them tries to climb inside. The catflap obsession has it's benefits. If you hear "tick, tick, tick" at least you know exactly what they are up to. It can still bring surprises like when they posted the kiwi through it.

Top tip: don't buy mountains of specialist "twin-proofing" gear upfront. Start with the basics once they start crawling: stair gates, and maybe a few cupboard locks, and then add to it depending on what kind of chaos your pair prefer. For example, we dutifully bought cupboard locks but haven't needed them so far. Every house (and every child) is different, and you can't predict everything. Paul for example in the past week is obsessed with investigating inside the toilet but shows no interest in cupboards. It was not for another three months that cupboards became a fascinating objective. Also, accept that some chaos is inevitable, sometimes it's quicker to clean up the carnage than to stop it happening in the first place.

The humble UK plug is a marvel of design. It is solid, safe, and brilliantly thought through. It can only ever be live if the earth pin (the big one at the top) is pushed in first, which in turn opens the shutters to the live and neutral. That means, by design, little fingers can't just poke into danger. Ironically, those brightly coloured plastic plug covers that are often sold as "childproofing" do the exact opposite. They bypass the safety mechanism and can actually make it easier for children to reach the live parts. The plug is safe and you do not need to buy any covers as part of your childproofing mission.

Managing outings solo or with help

Taking two babies out, especially if you're on your own, feels like a full military operation. Bags packed, snacks prepped, buggy folded, naps and feeds timed with precision… honestly, it's less like a quick walk to the park and more like planning a small expedition.

When you're solo-parenting, you quickly learn to plan routes with military precision too. No awkward steps, no narrow pavements especially if it is bin day, and definitely no buses without ramps. The number of times I've had to reverse out of a shop because the double buggy wouldn't fit is beyond a joke. On the other hand, when both of us are out together, it's like having a full support crew, one of us wrangles a boy while the other sorts snacks, directions, or buggy manoeuvres.

Top tip: always carry a spare top. For you, not just the babies. A milk spill, nappy leak, or overenthusiastic cuddle with sticky hands or snotty noses can derail your day faster than you'd think. When you're outnumbered, smelling like yoghurt isn't ideal. Cath's old old friends from secondary school treated us to a rucksack that now goes everywhere with us: nappies, wipes, an emergency bottle of formula with a sterile teat, spare clothes, hats, and all the regular essentials. More recently, it's evolved into a mobile tuck shop too, satsumas and breadsticks are our go-to emergency snacks.

Twinfinity and beyond: tornadoes to toddlerhood

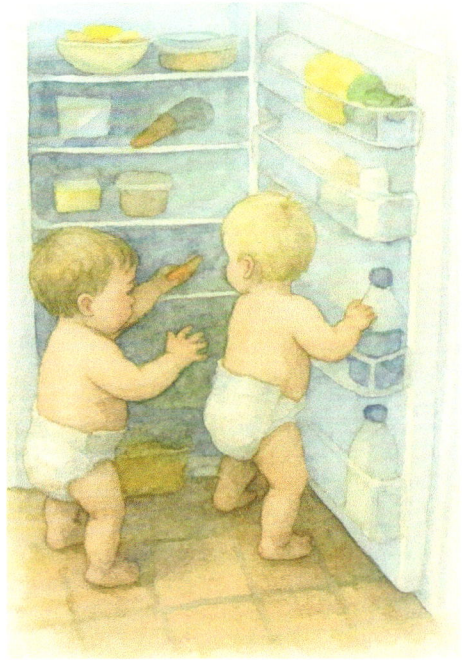

At first, I struggled to find a way to capture on paper what daily life with the twins really looks like. Then, one morning in France while on holiday, it hit me. Emma had started making little nature documentaries about fighting stag beetles and an incredibly rare Capricorn beetle we had spotted while walking around the lake. Those long, elegant antennae, their tiny armoured bodies... I couldn't help but hear David Attenborough narrating every movement.

Then suddenly, that's exactly how I saw our household with twins: a tiny, bustling ecosystem, full of strange behaviours and endless curiosity. Take Paul, for example. Watching him at any given moment, I can't help but think of him as roughly on the same evolutionary level as *Homo heidelbergensis* whose tools we can still find that were made half a million years ago. Give him a syringe, and he's experimenting: testing whether he can use it in combination with another "tool," or figuring out the mechanics of how it works. Observing him is like watching early humans at Boxgrove, puzzling out the world entirely by trial, error, and a fair amount of noise.

Picture the scene, and if you can, imagine the voice…

The sun rises over the urban sprawl of Southampton, casting a soft glow through the curtains of a modest British household. Behind one particular door, muffled scuffling can be heard, followed by a series of small, chaotic thuds. Then, emerging triumphantly with a cheeky grin, is one of two young juvenile males. Identical in appearance, but entirely different in temperament, the pair are already locked in their daily struggle for dominance… and survival.

Observe the food raid. The younger of the two juveniles leans across the highchair divide, one arm fully outstretched, fingers reaching as far as they can. He pilfers a nectarine slice as though it were the last of its kind on Earth. His brother protests with an indignant squeal. Such skirmishes are not uncommon in the day-to-day lives of these two spirited individuals. Sharing remains a concept as yet unmastered.

Later, we return to discover the elder of the two nibbling on a soft, malleable giraffe. A fine local delicacy known as Sophie. She has become the centre of a long-standing power struggle. The younger sibling, eager to reclaim her, now brandishes a mighty sceptre: the soft-bristled hairbrush. Once intended for gentle grooming, it is now the prize of whichever twin prevails in the ongoing toy-based conflict. Echoes, perhaps, of the ancient tale of Romulus and Remus, though mercifully with less bloodshed.

But not all is chaos. One of the juveniles has stepped away from the endless cycle of bashing and grabbing and turned instead to curious experimentation. Watch as a simple Calpol syringe is repurposed, transformed into a primitive tool. With great focus, he uses it to push a cardboard box across the floor. Success only comes when the syringe is used the correct way round. An early sign of engineering instinct in its rawest form.

Upon achieving this victory, the syringe is posted ceremoniously through the open top flap of a cereal box, its fate uncertain. It may never be seen again.

An emerging culture is taking shape. Both juveniles have discovered a passion for music. A saucepan, turned upside down, and a wooden spoon become the instruments for an improvised percussion session. There is no rhythm, no structure. What they lack in musicality, they more than make up for in volume and enthusiasm.

Now, as calm begins to settle over the sticky, chaotic ecosystem they call home, an adult arrives. One by one, the boys are scooped up, writhing, protesting, and placed into a peculiar wheeled contraption known locally as a double pushchair. For it is naptime. And though the battle for Sophie la Girafe will no doubt resume in mere hours, for now, they must rest. They are, after all, on a remarkable journey….

Even at this age, they've already cultivated a wild variety of hobbies. Most involve eating, bashing, whacking, or experimenting with things that really shouldn't be going in their mouths. Spoiler alert: chicken poo doesn't taste great. Who knew? Not exactly a shocker, but still, apparently worth the attempt.

Then there's the catflap. We've met it before but for reasons known only to them, it is a source of endless entertainment. We have one that opens only for the cat's microchip, and the boys love nothing more than flicking the lock. You can hear the "tick, tick, tick, tick" of tiny fingers at work as they faff about, utterly delighted. Our neighbour's catflap, sealed shut, has proved just as fascinating. Every time they spot it, they're determined to break through, only to end up disappointed.

Aside from infiltration attempts, their main obsession is noise. If a toy can be shaken, bashed, or activated to make noise, it's fair game. There's a particular cow toy that Cath despises in her sleep deprived state, and therefore they play with it constantly. It is almost as though they know exactly how much it winds her up.

Swimming was another milestone. Their first dip was at our friends Amanda and Kit's house, fitting, since Amanda herself has twins who are now in their fifties now. The boys were enthralled, staring at the shimmering water as if they'd just discovered a new planet. The novelty soon wore thin once they had become overstimulated with by new activity, but as we swam more, whether at Bluestone or abroad, they became water babies through and through. Chris throws himself headlong into shallow pools like he's auditioning for a stunt team, while Paul prefers the lazy river on a float, bobbing serenely like a miniature emperor on parade. In France, we even bought them an inflatable cactus. Chris immediately treated it like a mosh pit prop, headbanging manically against its side while cackling with glee. Thankfully, it wasn't prickly and I get the feeling like he is going to *love* Metal and our keyworker at the nursery agrees making suggestions for fun songs to introduce them to.

They first started properly crawling at Bluestone when they were eight months old. What had been tentative crawling had now transformed into lightning speed across any available surface. Paul, in particular, has proven himself a determined little character. My cousin's twins were of the sedentary variety, strolling into the world at seventeen and nineteen months, but Paul seems intent on hitting these milestones much earlier, each one a declaration of independence. Chris, by contrast, is often so busy with his own adventures that he barely registers the significance of taking steps, yet the moment he does, it opens whole new worlds for him… and, naturally, new stress levels for us.

Watching Paul wobble forward, stubbornly upright, is both thrilling and terrifying; one minute he's cruising toward a toy, the next he's heading straight for a sharp corner or a precariously stacked pile of books.

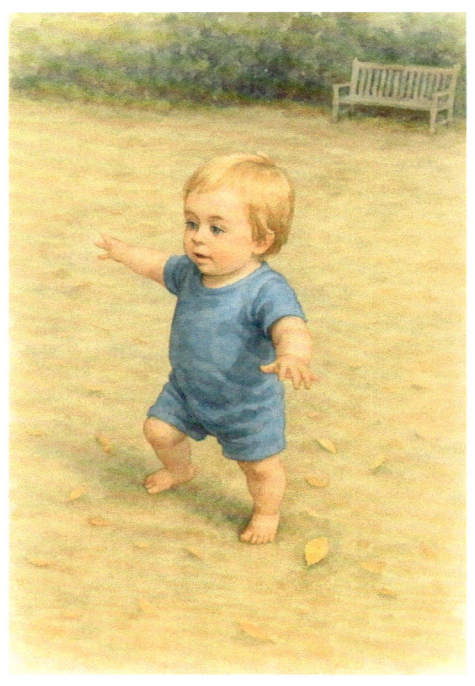

And then, of course, came the long-awaited spectacle: Paul's first steps. Unlike the graceful, tentative wobble one might expect, he moved sideways with a peculiar, scuttling gait, imagine a tiny crab negotiating the high seas of the living room carpet. At times, he resembled a miniature Dr. Zoidberg from *Futurama*, lab coat replaced with a T-shirt and trousers, claws replaced by chubby little hands flailing for balance. When I shared this triumph with my colleague Emma, herself a seasoned twin parent, her response was characteristically succinct: "You're %$&@£*." She understood instantly, the crab-walk was only the beginning. This sideways shuffle marked the start of a whole new chapter of chaos, exploration, and the slow, inexorable takeover of every flat surface in the house.

The next day Paul managed a few glorious, tentative and wobbly steps in a straight line towards Emma. One of my favourite moments was Paul walking on the green outside our house with Cath hovering behind him like a nervous yet proud bodyguard. He promptly toppled backwards and applauded himself, as if to say, *thank you, thank you, you've been a wonderful audience*. I had the camera rolling, certain we were about to capture history. The look on Cath's face watching this is probably what I like most about this moment.

But of course, Chris couldn't let his brother have the spotlight. He shot past on all fours crawling at Max *Wiss Speed*, completely upstaging the moment, and was already heading for the gravel buffet. Cath, forced to abandon Paul's standing ovation, had to swoop in before Chris could add "stoney snack" to his daily menu. Paul's first proper steps may have been monumental, but thanks to Chris, they'll forever be remembered as the warm-up act.

The current battleground fought over every day is a plastic walker. Chris loves it, so of course Paul wants it too. We do have another one, but it's wooden and heavier, which means naturally they both fight over the lighter one. I've even had to add tape to the wheels so it can be manoeuvred on the bumpy green outside. Thankfully our neighbours Rob and Emily had a spare they gave to use which meant we avoided *Twinzilla vs. Twin Kong*. Watching Chris attempt a 48-point turn with one of the walkers is basically the Austin Powers roller scene, only in toddler slow motion, with extra dribble.

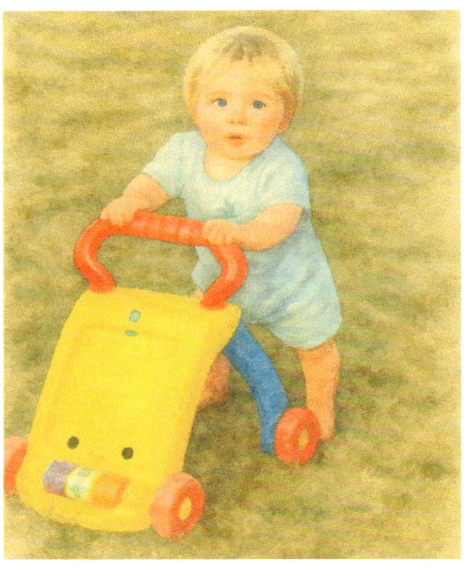

Watching Chris attempt a 48-point turn with one of the walkers is basically the Austin Powers roller scene, only in toddler slow motion, with extra dribble.

Paul was happily demolishing a satsuma watching the events unfold until he decided the Bugaboo push chair would make a better walker. Cue him crawling and shoving it along, grinning like he'd just invented the wheel until it went a bit too fast and he went face first into the grass.

Eventually one of them tipped the lighter walker over, and that's when science class began. They crouched, spun the wheels, flipped it upside down, testing why it no longer worked. For a moment, they weren't babies, they were hominids in transition, somewhere between *Homo heidelbergensis* and *Homo erectus*. Evolution in action, one wobbly step at a time. Next stop: cave painting. And given my "king of poo" moniker I award myself whenever an epic poo related catastrophe occurs, that frankly terrifies me.

Two become toddlers: chaos, joy and identity

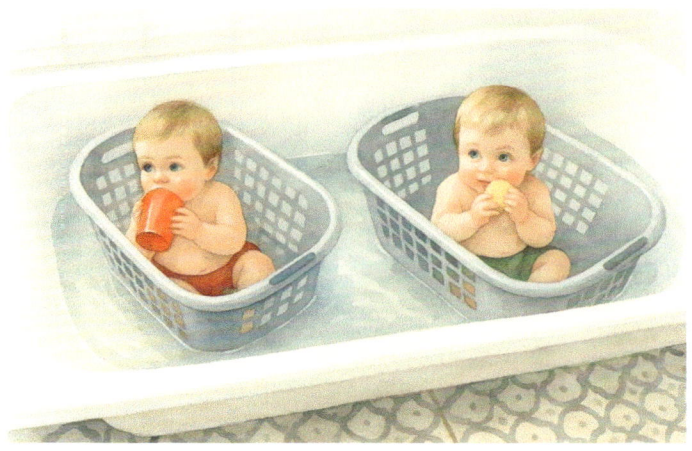

One real blessing, and I suspect many parents of multiples would agree, is that although life with two babies can be exhausting, they always have an available playmate. Of course, that doesn't mean harmony reigns. At ten months, if they find something they like, they'll proudly hold it up to show you. *But they absolutely do not want you to take it.* Unfortunately, to their brother, that gesture looks exactly like "Here, have this!"

They've started to anticipate this misunderstanding and perhaps use it as an opportunity to torture each other. Chris, ever the strategist, will twist his whole body around to hide a prized piece of fruit behind him after flashing it in his brothers face. Paul, in turn, erupts with indignation, convinced he's being mocked. Misunderstandings can end in shrieks, wrestling matches, sulks or turning blue and passing out. They're learning, sometimes the hard way, what sharing actually means.

Yet, despite the squabbles, their bond is unmistakable. They light each other up. Bath time becomes a comedy double act especially when we placed them within washing baskets to provide a bit of protection: Chris splashing like he's in training for "full-time splasher" status, while Paul dissolves into giggles as he has discovered his willy.

Individuality vs Twin Bonding

This is the paradox of twins: two individuals, bound so tightly together that their identities are constantly being shaped by each other. From the outside, it can feel like you're always describing them as a unit. *The boys, the twins.* Yet within that, they're working furiously to carve out their own selves.

Chris is often the instigator, the explorer, the one who charges in headfirst (sometimes literally). Paul is more measured, more watchful, sometimes content to let Chris test the waters before he joins in. They rely on each other, but they're also already learning how to be their own people. As parents, we're forever juggling the act of encouraging togetherness while also giving them space to grow as individuals.

Obviously, the harmony never lasts. There are certain daily battlefields over very specific toys. No matter how many duplicates we provide, it never solves the problem. They just want whatever their brother currently has. It's less about the object itself and more about possession: if he's got it, it must be worth having.

Sophie la Girafe, of course, is a frequent cause of skirmishes. She is gnawed, tugged, paraded in victory, and wrestled over like some kind of prized relic. Even when two toys which are exactly the same are offered simultaneously they both lunge for the *same one*, as though the rubber giraffe in my right hand is somehow infinitely superior. I'm sure this is a familiar battlefield for most families, but with twins it feels like every tussle is magnified.

Speech, Milestones, and Comparisons

Twin parents will tell you there's a constant temptation to compare. Who walked first? Who talked first? Who can stack blocks higher without knocking them down? It's almost impossible not to notice the differences, especially when milestones arrive at different times.

For us, the boys have developed in leapfrogs. Paul tends to surge ahead in certain areas, with Chris usually a week or so behind. That was the case with standing, crawling, and now walking. But while Paul might reach these stages first, it's Chris who truly embraces the opportunities for ill-considered adventure. He's the one who tries to scale the stairs, attempts head-first exits from the decking, or launches into whatever activity looks most likely to give us a heart attack.

Chris has also pulled ahead in other areas. His pincer grip with thumb and forefinger arrived early, making him a master thief when it comes to pinching Sophie la Girafe. He also started babbling and producing words first. Both boys' first word, fittingly enough, was "Emma."

It's reassuring, because you realise they're both on track in their own way. But it can also be maddening, because you can't stop the mental scoreboard in your head from ticking over. The trick, I've found, is reminding yourself that parenting twins is not a race. It's more like a relay. Sometimes one carries the baton a little further; sometimes the other does.

In some ways, having an in-house yardstick is actually useful. As we mentioned it meant by having this direct comparator we could spot the issue with Paul's hearing much earlier. The downside, of course, is that the "comparator" is usually scurrying off on his next reckless adventure while we're still processing the last one.

Nursery, School, and Social Life

In recent weeks, we've noticed some fascinating changes, especially as the twins approach nursery age. Chris, in particular, has become remarkably self-aware. Over the past few months, he seems to have discovered more about himself. He has gone from a little baby who didn't necessarily realise his place in the world to someone who is becoming much more sentient. It's a strange but wonderful stage.

His growing self-awareness brings its own challenges. Separation anxiety has reared its head, not out of mischief or defiance, but because he recognises that we, Cath and I, are people he can trust ad turn to when the world feels scary or uncertain. It's a sign that your little baby is starting to truly become a person.

It's a delicate balance: on one hand, it's heartwarming to be the person your child instinctively seeks out for comfort; on the other, it's a reminder that your role can't just be the provider of a lap to sit on all day. There are other things to do, other responsibilities to juggle, and the tiny humans who once fit entirely in your arms are now asserting themselves.

We imagine this self-awareness is going to make the early days of nursery a little more challenging. One might picture a nervous, tearful baby being left for a few hours. What I suspect is more likely to happen is that shortly after arrival, boisterous and adventurous Chris will appear, climbing anything, exploring every box, posting anything important somewhere obscure that will only be found in a decade, and discovering every little mischievous opportunity for mischief.

Yet, this same adventurous, risk-defying little character will always come to you for comfort if he spots Zog, his cuddly toy. He is nervous of Zog and crawls to us and sits on our lap watching Zog intently just in case he decides Chris is a princess, *ROARS*, kidnaps him and then flies straight into a tree.

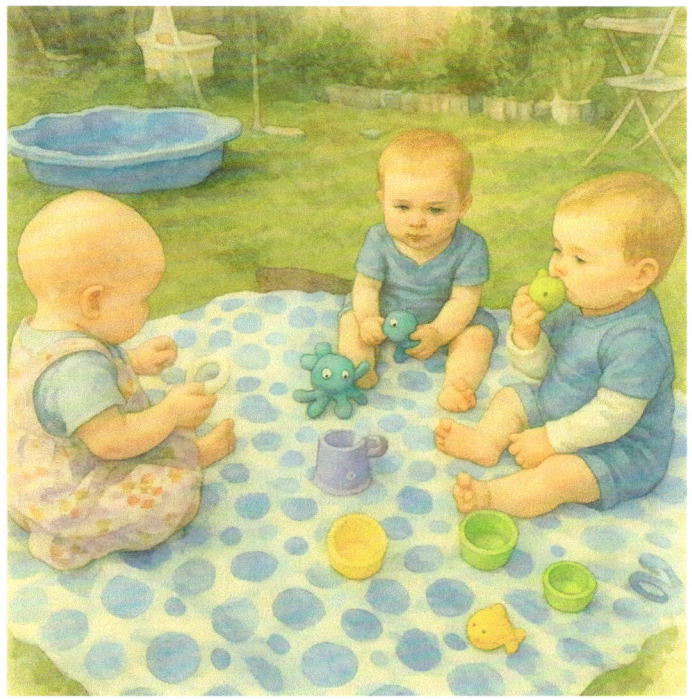

We've seen these changes not just in the boys, but in their friend Lucy too, who is only a few days older. It's been fascinating watching how the three of them have started to interact, their little personalities beginning to shine through. Recently, we even uncovered our first major scandal. The great pea heist. One of the trio (we're withholding names to protect the guilty) was caught red-handed, gleefully swiping peas from the high chair tray of a baby who was discovering gravity first hand. The look of sheer pride said it all. Crime clearly pays, at least when it comes to vegetables.

Holidays with twins

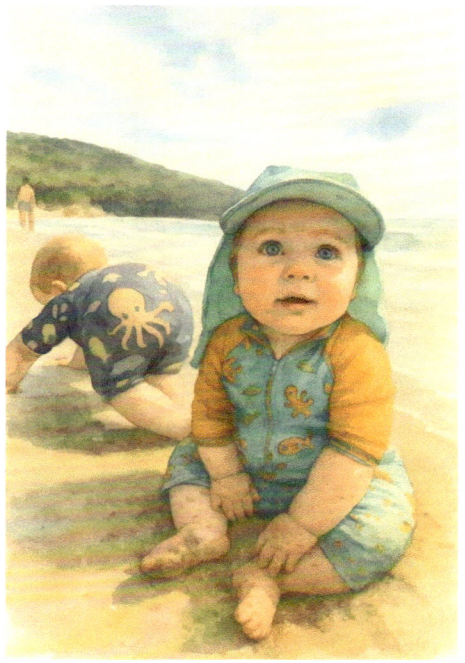

We decided to make the most of our parental leave, and the boys' relative immobility, by planning some trips. First up was Bluestone in Wales with my parents, Cath's parents, and their wider family. For Emma, this was wonderful, she had cousins to play with and endless activities to keep her entertained. Much of the time at home we were tied down with the twins, and she'd been incredibly patient and understanding. Now that the boys were starting to respond more, it was lovely for her to interact with them. At least until they inevitably damaged something she was working on, or tried to 'join in' a game by removing cards or letter tiles, at which point her enthusiasm tended to fade.

The second trip was on a rather grander scale. We travelled to Italy for the wedding of my former assistant, Cristina. It was an incredible holiday, but quite possibly one of the most stressful things I've ever organised. The chaos started before we even left the country, with the small matter of getting passports for the boys. Paul's was rejected three times because of his torticollis, which meant he couldn't quite hold his head at the regulation "neutral" angle required by His Majesty's Passport Office. On the fourth attempt, armed with a note from the osteopath, it was finally accepted. The result? Paul now officially travels the world with a passport photo that makes him look like he's posing for a jaunty album cover.

We'd anticipated that flying with twins would be challenging. On our type of aircraft, we couldn't all sit together, so I was a row ahead. Paul had fluid in his ear at the time, which a specialist had warned would make changes in pressure, especially on landing, quite uncomfortable. They were right.

Many aspects of the journey were manageable, helped by the fact that people seem to light up at the sight of twins, especially blonde-haired, blue-eyed ones. At Rome, we were even ushered into the VIP/diplomatic lane, ending up behind Rosamund Pike and her family. Paul who was clutching a very bright bag containing our passports, would not stop grinning at her spectacular hat. Sadly he did not get a smile back.

The real trouble began at the car hire desk in Italy. We'd booked a suitable vehicle well in advance, knowing we needed space for two car seats, Emma in the middle and a *lot* of luggage. The man behind the desk dropped a huge bombshell when he simply told us, "We don't have a car for you." His solution? A Fiat 500.

They offered an upgrade to a larger car for an extra €1,100. Unsurprising, given it was the first day of the English school half term. Everywhere was fully booked. I was stunned by how little the staff seemed to care that they were leaving a family with very young twins stranded three hours drive from our accommodation in a busy car park.

Cath, however, kept her cool and had an incredibly firm, yet polite, conversation with them. Miraculously, a car appeared. It wasn't ideal, but we could make do. Then came the next hurdle: they only had one car seat, and their "helpful" suggestion was to drive illegally with a twin on our lap to a local shopping mall to buy another. That was not going to happen.

We tried every other car hire desk for a second seat, most of which simply said "no" and moved on. Then Cath spoke to one man who, after learning his own son had been born the exact same day as our twins, disappeared for ten minutes and returned with a spare seat, free of charge, saying, "We trust you to bring it back." He saved our holiday. It still meant we arrived about three and a half hours late, but at least we were safe.

By contrast, the original car hire company left us sitting outside their office for hours without even acknowledging us. Watching Cath through the soundproof glass explaining that the situation was theirs to fix was the most intense look I've ever seen her give… One I hope never to receive myself.

When we finally reached our villa, it was stunning, a peaceful setting with a shared pool, shaded terraces, and hidden rooms some of us didn't discover for days. That first evening, we headed to the supermarket for supplies. The boys, having spent all day in either a plane or a car, revelled in the freedom of being wheeled around in two trolleys, grinning at everyone.

It was a rural shop and no one spoke English and my Italian is terrible but I knew the Italian word for "twins." Before long the bakery lady was calling "gemelli!" across to her colleagues at the delicatessen and meat counters. The boys were soon nibbling on schiacciata, a salty flatbread, which they loved.

Food had been an ongoing adventure since their six-month birthday, when we'd first introduced solids. The boys absolutely loved Italy, mainly for the sheer amount of pizza they could eat. We tried a few different pizzerias, including one in the defended village of Campagnatico, where they happily sat eating for ages. After about an hour, they got restless and wanted to get down onto the floor. Luckily, most Italians are very relaxed about children making a bit of a nuisance of themselves in restaurants. In this case, though, the boys didn't go wandering, instead, they shuffled around like little Labradors, hoovering up discarded offcuts from their own pizzas that they'd previously dropped. We are hopeful that this was good for their immune systems. What doesn't kill you…

The holiday was blissful but physically demanding. The villa's stone floors made it a dangerous playground for two babies suddenly keen to pull themselves up on everything as they were able to stand up properly for the first time. We were in Italy during the early heatwave in Europe, I often took them for long walks along the country lanes. 20,000 to 30,000 steps a day, in full sun, with no shade. It was the kind of thing only mad dogs and Englishmen would do, but it kept the twins content, me unexpectedly fit and I saw wolf cubs! When I got them back to the villa, my next step was to usually just jump in the pool.

Consuelo, the wonderful woman who managed the property, advised us to visit a beach called Cala Violina, near Scarlino, for the boys' very first seaside experience. It's named Cala Violina because if you walk along the sand, you can hear sounds that kind of resemble a violin playing under your feet. You can hear it when you walk until two fed up babies chime in.

In peak season, access is limited to just a couple of hundred people a day and you have to book a long way in advance, but since we were travelling in May, we were lucky enough for it to feel like we almost had the spot to ourselves.

It's a beautiful spot with endless corners for the boys to explore. They were mesmerised by the sea, standing for ages just watching it, half curious and half suspicious. Then suddenly Chris shouted "charge!", hurled himself straight in head first, and came out absolutely soaked. The shock of the cold took him by surprise, but he loved it all the same. For a first place to really discover the sea, it was a pretty special choice.

While Emma and I wandered along the beach in search of keepsakes, she picked up a piece of seaglass, and I found two smooth grey stones. Emma dismissed them out of hand but when wet you could see they were veined with glittering seams. On them I wrote: *our first visit to the sea*. Naturally, at the end of the day, this being Italy, every outing finished with gelato, the perfect closing note.

One of the most magical parts of visiting Tuscany, and later Cortona (where the wedding was taking place), was seeing fireflies. It was the first time I'd ever spotted them. The first one I saw, I honestly thought was just someone walking past smoking a cigarette as it was by the road. But then more and more appeared, until there were dozens twinkling in the dark. I was so excited to show Emma the next day, and the boys, when they were awake. You could tell they were trying to figure out what on earth they were looking at, as the fireflies didn't behave like anything they'd ever seen before.

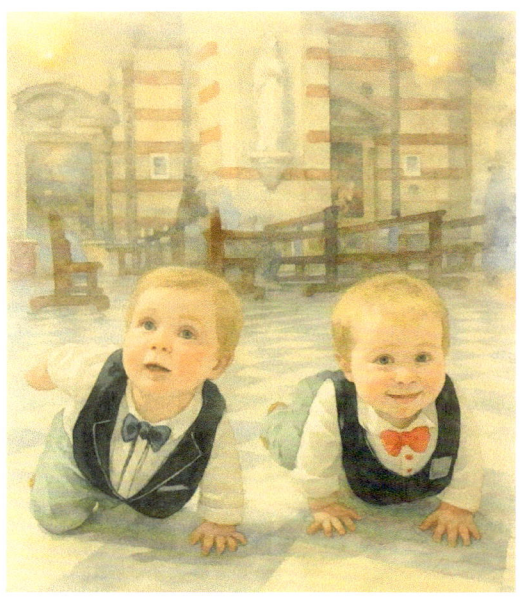

The wedding itself was wonderful, even if for large parts we had very little idea what was actually happening. The ceremony took place in the beautiful Basilica of Saint Margaret of Cortona, with views over the Italian landscape that looked like something from a painting. The boys wore tuxedo bibs, the perfect compromise between formality and dribble-resistance. We let them sit on the floor to quietly gnaw on their teethers, which seemed like the most peaceful solution, until a nun made it very clear that two babies sitting quietly on the floor was not acceptable.

Emma was in her element during the photos, which involved bubbles. She appointed herself chief bubble-blower and for the next two hours made sure no one within ten feet escaped without being showered. The reception was in a gorgeous vaulted hall where the boys happily crawled up and down between the rows of golden chairs before joining in the dancing with the live rock and roll band. Watching two babies bum wiggle along to Elvis was not something we had expected from the day, but it was a highlight all the same.

One thing I find really interesting is how different countries react to twins. As soon as we landed in Italy, people were absolutely buzzing to see the boys. You could hear all sorts of excited shouts of "Gemelli! Twins!" everywhere. From airport security to random passersby. Most people (car hire companies excluded here) went out of their way to help us. Italians love children especially blonde haired blue eyed double trouble.

By contrast, over in France, the reaction was a bit different. Everyone was really friendly, but it was probably the only place where we didn't get quite the same level of excitement about the twins. In England, people stop you daily to ask about them. In France, for at least the first week, people would smile kindly, like the lady who ran the local shop, but there wasn't that same unbridled enthusiasm where strangers who can't speak English just stop you in the street, desperate to have a look.

In France, we hit a triple whammy of poorly, teething and unsettled boys. Cue nonstop ibuprofen and paracetamol all day, horrible teething pain, and, unsurprisingly, some truly dreadful nappies. The poor little guys were really upset. On top of that, Chris suddenly developed some serious separation anxiety. There were moments when we had to take one baby somewhere to try and help them feel better, and the other would just scream like the world was ending. It made doing anything nearly impossible because Chris would get upset so quickly.

At the same time, it was crucial to meet Emma's needs and expectations. She wanted to do things like tackle a GoApe-style zip line course across the lake, try out the Total Wipeout inflatables, hunt for kingfishers while making nature documentaries, or simply play air hockey at the arcade. Balancing all of that with the twins' care was tricky. It usually required careful planning on our part, booking key activities for times when the twins were likely to be asleep or content in the buggy. Finding those pockets of time ensured Emma didn't feel she was missing out, which was essential for her enjoyment (the 'FOMO' strikes young!).

As importantly, Cath was finding the nights brutal because the boys were poorly. It was important to also ensure she could get some peace. She happily signed up for three yoga sessions for some self-care. Emma joined the first one and was bored... she spent the next hour huffing at the back of the class.

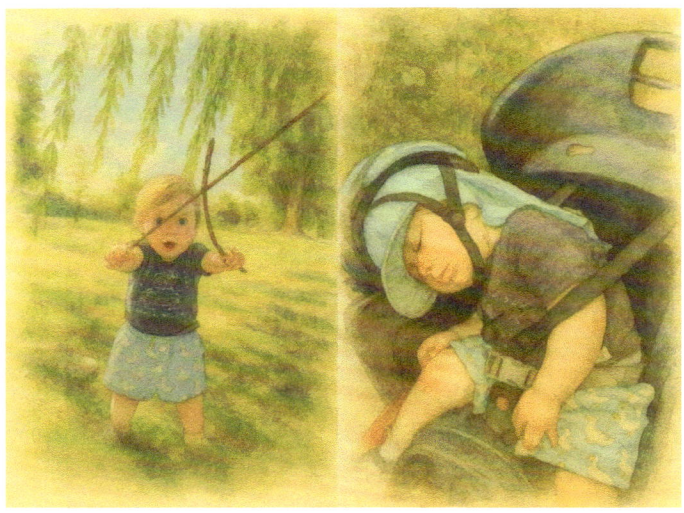

While it was challenging for us, and there were even moments when we talked about going home early when the boys were so poorly. There were also some wonderful memories. One of my favourites was a simple cycle ride to the local town. Our first proper family bike outing with the boys in toddler seats. Their reactions were mixed: Paul hated wearing his helmet but loved the "outrageous" speeds (maybe 10 mph!) as we descended the hill.

Along the way, there was so much to see, fields of sunflowers, quaint village scenes, and a beautiful lake. Paul amused himself by playing with sticks as if they were dowsing rods, searching for water, and he was clearly successful, as the lake was right there. Chris, meanwhile, was full of excitement, giggling about going on adventures no one had dared before. Before promptly falling asleep in his seat. It was such a joy to share this simple outing together as a family.

Tips for Travelling with Twins & Emergency Kit

I thought I was pretty well prepared with a medicine kit for trips away from home, two bottles of ibuprofen, two of paracetamol, various syringes (since the hard ones aren't always popular with the boys), nappy bags, and other bits and bobs.

We ended up realising there were still many bits we needed. Some were unexpected such as Chris needed some attention after rubbing himself in the eye with an apricot. Unsurprisingly, it was very sticky! Others, such as a tick twister, we only realised after they played on a lawn.

It really is best to be well prepared with twins, and I had been making an emergency car kit stored in our boot. It grew from a mini first-aid stash with scissors, plasters, cotton buds, water wipes, and a few other essentials. Knowing we have this kit means we're covered even if we get cut short or need something quickly. We also keep a couple of spare IKEA bibs in the car, along with spare clothes for both the boys and Emma, in case of particularly messy incidents. These days we have other additions such as nail clippers and a sewing kit.

Travelling top tips

Pack duplicates of everything you *might* need if you can: From nappies and wipes to bibs and favourite snacks. It sounds excessive but we discovered nappies abroad were much more expensive. All the Italian wipes we found in the smaller shops were also heavily fragranced.

Always have an emergency kit for the car: There will always be new things you need be it a tick twister or more bibs.

Prepare for food adventures: Even picky babies sometimes surprise you. While both boys loved the fruit and vegetables, pizza in France for example just did not appeal.

Expect stress and delays: Especially with car hire or flights. but remember the holiday is for everyone, and calm parents help calm babies.

Don't underestimate the joy of simple things: Pools, beaches, fireflies, and ice cream will delight twins as much as adults. It creates memories (some of) you will never forget.

Finding our balance (or at least trying to)

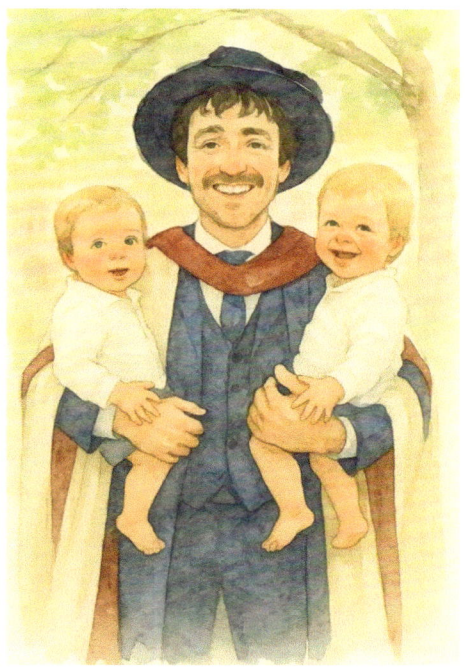

I'd submitted my doctoral thesis just a couple of months before the boys were born. To earn a PhD, you have to endure a *viva voce*, three hours of interrogation, dressed up as intellectual conversation. Not the sort of ordeal you want to face the morning after your babies have been freshly vaccinated and determined that no one in the house should sleep.

Still, there was an unexpected blessing in having finished when I did. It means I work part time and could be present for moments I might otherwise have missed, had I been juggling long commutes or endless travel. Given how spectacular some stages were, and others spectacularly difficult, some were precious, some were just survival. For Cath, it also meant I could help out a lot, especially when she was running on empty.

I got to see those lightning-fast developmental changes that can happen in less than a week. Of course, the boys seemed to reserve their biggest leaps for the least convenient, least safe locations possible. They learned to crawl while we were on holiday in Wales. They learned to stand in Italy, unfortunately, without learning how to get back down again safely. If you're going to practise standing in a place where every floor is tiled or stone, you can expect plenty of bumps and tears.

By the time we went camping in France for a couple of weeks, we half-expected them to start walking. We even bought shoes, assuming that if a new skill came with an added risk factor, it would happen far from the padded safety of home. In reality our estimates were one week off and Paul took his first steps the week after we got back.

Financially, two part-time incomes can be tricky, especially in those last few months of Cath's maternity leave, when we were living on statutory pay or nothing. But we decided to make the most of it with a string of holidays. It's harder for Cath to take long breaks now; as a vet, her job can literally be life or death, and there always needs to be a certain number of vets on site. My work, by contrast, involves caring for dead things, very old and very dead things, in a museum. There are deadlines and exhibition schedules, yes, but nothing quite as urgent as a patient on the operating table.

As well as being a museum curator, I do freelance work writing up assemblages of coins and objects from different sites across Britain. In the rest of the non-existent free time I have I also write books and research publications and try to run a woodworking business.

Trying to do all that while finishing off corrections for parts of my PhD with two babies in tow was, frankly, quite the challenge at first. In the first few weeks, it wasn't too bad because the boys were so small. You could have them snoring away, resting on your shoulders, happily staying like that for an hour or so. Now they're much bigger, and you can't really do that anymore. When they're tired, they just don't sleep the same way.

I still think about the Roman coin identification book I wrote. I often had Paul on my right shoulder and Chris on my left, trying to do bits of Photoshop or make amendments whenever I could grab half an hour here and there. It was easier as they would simply fall asleep and lie there curled up in the foetal position.

Writing this book, for example, has been tricky. Since we have to go on so many long walks to get the boys to sleep, we tried dictating. That didn't always work out brilliantly. When I was going through the Apple notes, Paul was spelt correctly about 95% of the time, when it was wrong it had typed Wade, I am still not sure why. Throughout Chris was misspelt as Kris. And trying to dictate complicated medical terms? Let's just say they came out all sorts of ways that made it tricky to decipher what I was actually trying to say.

As well as secretly having a third child called Wade through the wonders of dictation, it's also been a bit of a challenge to translate at times. I dictated quite a lot of this text while walking around a beautiful lake at a campsite in France. Each lap took about 20 minutes, and I reckon I completed 75-100 loops. Firstly that is a lot of notes to go through... Secondly you end up with dictation that's peppered with other people's conversations. Just now it's got loads of chat about fishing thrown in. There are also random "bonjour"'s and "hello"'s popping up throughout.

While it was useful to get something down quickly, I imagine no editor would be thrilled with the resulting draft. It certainly has taken a lot of time to polish and make sense of what on earth I was talking about at the time as much of it I was living on just an hour or twos sleep.

While I was attempting to see whether it was humanly possible to juggle a PhD, a museum job, freelance projects, a woodworking business, and twins, Cath's maternity leave came to an end. The result was the kind of logistical puzzle you might set in an escape room: two parents working, two babies not yet in nursery, and roughly zero spare hands. Thursdays were our main problem as it was a day we both had to be in.

We spent ages debating whether to go for a nursery, or have a nanny. The nanny was tempting, after all, the boys could stay home most of the day, and there were other perks, but in the end we decided that a nursery made more sense. Partly because it let us use the free childcare hours, and partly because being officially registered meant we could access childcare vouchers. It's a bit of a complicated system. You have to register every quarter or you lose out, but in the long run it's going to be massively helpful, letting us squeeze a couple of extra workdays in than we had expected.

The tricky part was that when we initially enquired, the nursery said there were no spaces until October and Cath was going back to work in the middle of August... We were very lucky that they managed to fit us in early, even though taking two at once, especially in the same room, can be tricky. To bridge this gap I ended up doing the bulk of the childcare myself, using up all my leave.

That meant August and September became "Daddy Daycare Month," where I was on duty from around 7 am until 7 pm every Thursday. Brutal? Yes.

On Cath's first day back at work I woke up tired but optimistic: I could do this. I was in charge. Nothing would go wrong. I'd looked after the boys on long days before, but never for a whole month. I could look after them by myself. Everything would be fine.

Then came the morning chaos. Paul's nappy was full to bursting, the kind that should come with a warning label. Halfway through changing him, I noticed something alarming: Chris had discovered that he could put his hand in his nappy. And, of course, he decided to share his discovery by stroking Paul's stomach.

That wasn't the end. Chris then investigated his own feet and legs, before turning his attention to one of his toys: a wooden cog board. Normally, the boys can take the cogs off and slot them back on, and when they're all in place, moving one cog sets the whole lot spinning in a beautifully satisfying chain reaction. Today, however, poo was blocking the cogs. They refused to spin. The toy became sticky and stubborn, taking ages to clean. Baby hand prints, smeared toys, and chaos spread across the living room like some abstract modern-art installation. The poo situation was so bad I ended up washing Chris in the sink.

Normally, this would be just a messy blip. But today was different. This was my first solo stretch of full-time parenting for a month, and we had a very important medical appointment at 8:30. Breakfast hadn't even happened yet, and Chris's favourite hobby these days is trying to escape his seat rather than eat. I had no room for poo-led disasters or challenging breakfast chaos.

Looking after both boys alone is a military operation where failure isn't an option. One lapse, and you're staring down a full-scale poopocalypse. A few days later, on a 12-hour shift that began at 7.30 a.m., the inevitable struck again. The fallout was catastrophic: clothes ruined, toys destroyed, books lost to the brown tide, and poor Chris covered from ears to toes by his own wandering hands. There were no survivors, only bleach and a drowned rat post impromptu sink bath. The books were from the 'that's not my' series which have tactile surfaces. Thanks to Chris, *That's not my car* could have become *that is my poo!*

It's easy to feel defeated. On the outside, I may have looked calm, but underneath I was paddling like a swan on steroids. And yet… even in chaos, you're raising two, even when its hard you have to remember you're doing a fantastic job.

Parenting twins will slap your confidence around, smear it in unexpected places, and leave you wondering if you'll ever be in control again. But it's also ridiculous. It's funny. And when you survive the epic fails, you realise that surviving at all is winning.

Some days, a sink bath for a toddler counts as a victory. Some days, the only thing you can do is laugh, mop up, and remember that you've earned your crown back, at least until the next round of nappy roulette. Unfortunately, despite my best efforts, I am still the King of Poo in the household.

While navigating daddy day care and the ongoing poopocalypse, I still had to somehow carve out a day and a half of work each week to stop all the plates I had spinning from crashing down. That meant museum responsibilities, keeping freelance projects alive, staying on top of proofs and editorial deadlines for articles and books, and, because I thought it was a good idea at the time, continuing to build up stock for Christmas markets with my woodworking.

Trying to do all of that on two hours' sleep a night, even after eleven months, was a kind of madness I don't think you can fully describe. Everything took three times longer than it should, and every small job felt like climbing a mountain. I'd often be sanding chopping boards in the evening or setting up a coin catalogue at midnight, long after both boys had finally given in and gone to sleep. The following morning, it was straight back into nappies, bottles, and damage control.

There were moments when it all felt almost comical. I even decided to write a letter to Sir David Attenborough, complete with a printout of our very own "nature documentary" on the twins from an earlier chapter. Chris promptly stole the first sheet of the letter, while Paul started teething on my fountain pen. We did get a reply, sort of. One morning I spotted our stamped, self-addressed envelope lying on the floor and felt a surge of excitement. But when I picked it up, it was damaged and completely empty.

If Chris hadn't been napping at the time, I would have strongly suspected him as the culprit. So, I wrote again (I'm nothing if not persistent. Think Andy Dufresne from *The Shawshank Redemption*). Wonderfully, instead of a cease and desist letter that I was half expecting I got a reply from the 99 year old national treasure hoping the book was proceeding well.

There were times I'd be replying to an academic email about Roman coin distributions with one hand while holding a wriggling baby with the other determined to eat the power cable, restocking my shelf of items on sale at October Books with grizzly babies demanding more orange slices or trying to pack Etsy orders while singing nursery rhymes about currant buns to keep the boys entertained.

The reality was that "work-life balance" wasn't really balance at all. It was more like frantic juggling while being pelted with half-chewed breadsticks.

While I was wrestling with dictation software and deadlines, Cath was navigating an entirely different kind of balance. Returning to work meant swapping twin chaos for the frenetic pace of vetting. A lot of coffee was consumed! I was grateful to be able to use some annual leave to return to work on reduced hours while Richard was doing the majority of twin-care. The lack of a continuous sleep-cycle at night meant I was never hitting the ground running but it was great to be back working with the awesome team at Chris Carter's. After two weeks back I had a few days off to help ease Emma back into her new school year after a double inset day during which we happily spent a day at Splashdown with her cousin Peter.

The mental load: surviving and thriving as twin parents

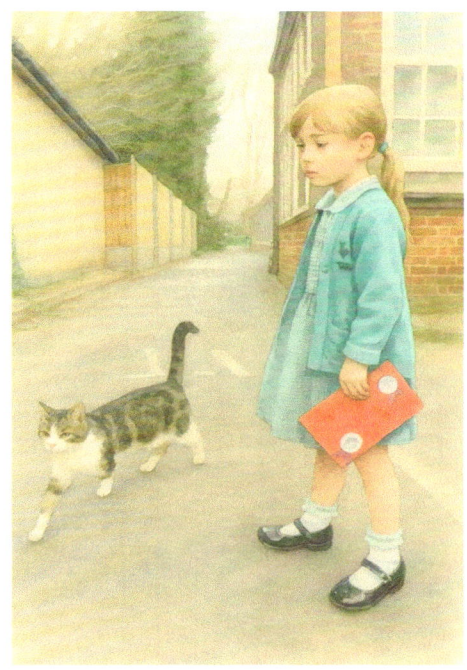

Something I don't think I fully appreciated before was just how much these two would reshape not only their identity, but ours as well. It reminds me of when Emma first started school and we had a cat called Pip, a fearless little adventurer with more curiosity than road sense.

Pip had this habit of wandering into Emma's school, sometimes padding straight into classrooms or even appearing in the dinner hall as if she were on the register. Nobody could quite figure out what she was up to, but from then on Emma became "the owner of Pip the cat." Her whole identity, at least in that school community, was wrapped up in this cheeky animal.

Sadly, Pip's bold streak didn't mix well with traffic, and she died much younger than we'd hoped (racing through her nine lives much too quickly). But even now, if you ask anyone who was at that school, they'll still remember Pip, the classroom-crashing cat who somehow managed to become everyone's mascot.

In a strange way, twins have done something similar to us. Wherever we go now, people know us as "the parents of Chris and Paul, the twins." It's not Richard the curator, researcher, or writer anymore or Cath the researcher, teacher or vet. Those roles are still there, but they're now framed around the all-encompassing job of being parents to Double Trouble. The staff in Waitrose, Sainsbury's, and the post office always stop to ask how the boys are doing.

One of the strange things about having twins is how many different people end up having an affinity with them: friends, family, random strangers or the wonderful staff at Waitrose. It can feel a bit much sometimes, like everyone has a tiny claim on them. But I actually love seeing how people get excited watching them grow, from these tiny, spooky little babies into the cheeky, lively boys they are today. Now, when we're out and about, there are plenty of familiar faces who know them by sight, and hopefully the boys are a little bit cheeky back, grinning and greeting everyone like the little characters they've become. Around Southampton, faces light up when they spot the double buggy with its pink and purple bird-patterned hoods, and everyone seems to know what's inside.

On the Common, it can feel a bit like a parade. People stop to tell us about their own twins, about siblings who are twins, or about grown-up children who once used to share a buggy just like ours. It's heart-warming, but it also makes you realise how much your sense of self changes once you're parents. Strangers expect to see the babies with us, and if they're not, there's often a puzzled or even disappointed reaction. Once upon a time, I could walk through town and blend into the crowd. Now I feel more like I'm part of a travelling exhibit: *"Here come the twins!"*

And identity doesn't just shift in how others see you, it shifts in how you see yourself. My world used to more heavily defined by work deadlines and research projects as well as spending time with Cath and Emma. Now, while I still write, curate, and research, the bulk of my time and identity is shaped much more by family: looking after Chris and Paul, supporting Cath, and also being there for Emma. Watching her grow into such a thoughtful and kind young woman is something I am deeply proud of. I may not be her father, but in every way that matters she feels like the daughter I was never destined to have, and the best one someone could ever wish for. I guess that this is a change everyone experiences when they become a parent.

Of course, we're already thinking about how identity works for the boys, too. Other parents of twins have told us that once they hit their teens, twins often want to be seen as individuals, not just as a matched set. We can understand why, growing up with someone who knows you inside out is a gift, but it's also a challenge when you want to step out and be recognised for *yourself*. For now, Chris and Paul are inseparable, partners in crime who share everything from toys to tantrums, but we're conscious of how important it will be to let them develop as individuals as they grow.

And then there are the smaller identity-shaping moments, the little connections we make with people because of them. Trevor, our postie, is a good example. He always waves when he sees me on yet another marathon nap walk, stops to chat with Emma, and genuinely seems invested in how the boys are doing. One day, Chris was crying like the world was ending while dressed in a fluffy suit that made him look like a furious teddy bear. Trevor came over, clearly worried. In reality, all that had happened was that a leaf had landed on Chris's face, an ordinary oak leaf from the Common. To him, it was a catastrophe. To me, it was so comically disproportionate that I had to take a photo. So now I've got this picture of an angry little bear with a leaf on his head, while Trevor looks on with genuine concern before laughing when I told him the disaster that had struck.

As I write this, Chris is starting to grumble again. I'd better check there isn't an oak leaf lurking nearby.

Most of the time we really are in tune as parents, and that's been the mainstay of what's kept us such a tight unit. There are ups and downs, of course, but the default has always been working together rather than pulling apart. When one of us is exhausted, the other steps in. When one is overwhelmed, the other steadies things. That rhythm doesn't happen by accident; it's been built in the small, ordinary choices we make every day.

Keeping our relationship alive in the middle of everything has taken effort, but not the kind of grand gestures people often imagine. It's been about the small things. Sitting outside together with a coffee before the chaos of the day kicks off, even if it's only for five minutes. Buying each other little gifts, not diamond necklaces or anything glamorous, but a slice of cake picked up because the day had been tough, or a small thing spotted in a shop that just felt "so you." Those gestures, tiny as they were, became anchors. They said, "I see you, and I've got you," at times when words would have been too heavy.

We've also made Fridays something of a sacred space. Both of us have the day off, and I've tried to keep it as clear as possible, because that time is precious. It's the one day of the week where we're not pulled in different directions by work or endless to-do lists, and we can actually spend time together. Sometimes that looks like catching up on life admin, but often it's just about being alongside each other without interruption. In a season of life where every moment feels scheduled, those Fridays feel like a pocket of breathing space we both really treasure.

We've learned that resilience hasn't come from big breakthroughs or dramatic changes, but from the rituals and routines we quietly stitched into daily life. The moments of laughter when the boys do something ridiculous, the little nods of encouragement when we're both on the edge, the unspoken understanding of when to step in or when to step back. All those things add up. They keep the wheels turning, and more than that, they keep us together.

There have been personal ups and downs too. Times when we've both felt like we've lost touch with the people we used to be. It's easy to forget yourself when every waking minute is filled with nappies, naps, feeds, and keeping small humans alive. Also, we are human, we do not always get it right so there are sharp words said often because when you have been living off two hours sleep a night tempers can fray.

Life with double trouble. How to survive being a big sister to twins – By Emma (8)

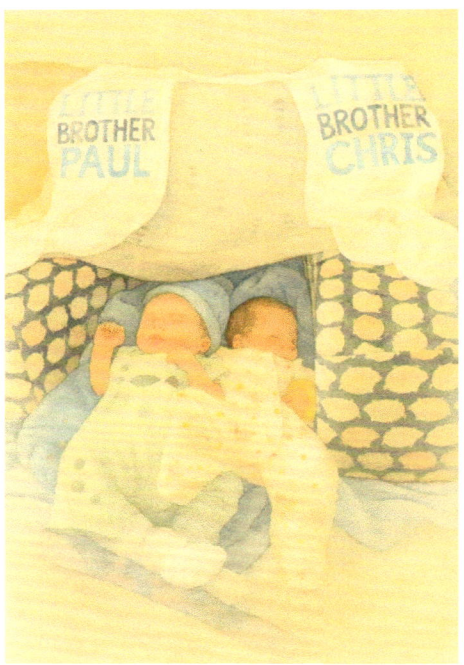

When I first found out there were going to be two babies, not just one, I was so surprised. The first thing I asked was if they were boys or girls. Then Mum showed me the scan pictures, and there were five of them that looked like there were six babies in there. I was like, "Wait... are we having six babies?!" Everyone laughed so much at that.

I kind of hoped for girls because I thought they might be a bit less rough. But then I thought, if they were girls, they'd probably grow up and steal all my stuff. So I didn't really mind either way.

When I found out I was getting twin brothers, I was so excited. Mostly because I thought it would be fun to play with them, and because there would be two new people in the family. And it is fun… most of the time.

I was a bit nervous too. I worried about the noise they'd make, how much poo there'd be, and whether they'd bash everyone. To get ready for them, I even asked my older friend Mai for advice. She told me, very seriously, "Panic!" I didn't actually panic, but it made me laugh and helped me feel less nervous.

At school, I took the scan pictures in for show and tell. That's when you bring something special into class and tell everyone about it, like a favourite toy, a pet, or, in my case, my brand-new twin brothers. Not many people even knew I had twin brothers yet, so it was fun to tell them. My two best friends' minds were totally blown. Livvy just kept saying how rare twins are, and Millie was so happy. She said, "It's not every day your best friend gets two baby brothers at once."

Watching Mum's tummy get bigger and bigger was so weird. It was hard to understand, because I didn't really know what to expect. I kept guessing when they'd arrive. In my head, I really wanted them to come on the first of October so that all our birthdays would be around the same time.

The day before Mum and Richard went into the hospital, I helped get the boys' room ready. We set it all up, put their new clothes away, and I made a little den out of my snuggly toys and some cushions. We put a lamp in there so it felt cosy. Richard and I made a mobile together too. It had sea creatures like a dolphin, a whale, jellyfish, and a shark, plus some little boats, and it spun around. When the boys were a bit older, they used to stare at it for ages, even when it wasn't moving, just because of all the colours. We're planning to make glow-in-the-dark things for their room too – stars, suns, and maybe even planets.

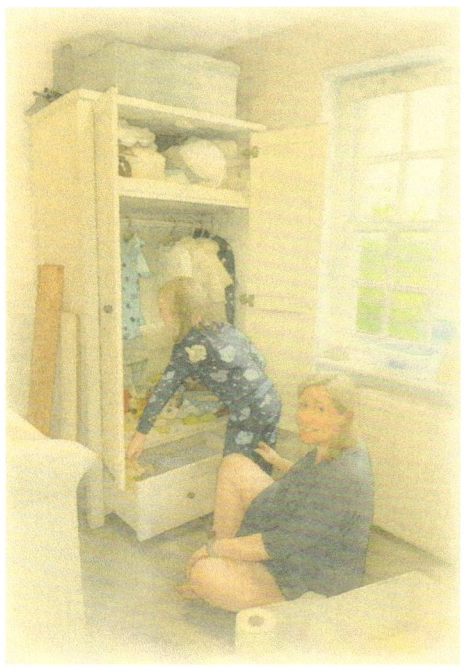

I spent a lot of time imagining what they'd look like, but I was completely wrong. I thought they'd have dark brown hair like Mum's and brown eyes. Instead, they've got blonde hair and blue eyes. I also thought they'd be completely identical and we'd never be able to tell them apart, but they aren't.

While Mum and Richard were still in the hospital, I got to have sleepovers on a school night. I stayed in the spare room at Millie's house. It was really fun, but I was so happy to come home when Mum and the boys did.

When I first met them in the hospital, I was so excited. I had my "Big Sister" T-shirt on and everything. Nana and Papa took me to see them. I even made them a little fort to sit in, but Mum told me to take the top off so it wouldn't fall on them while they were sleeping.

When they were really tiny, I loved holding them, even though I was a little nervous. They were so small, and it only took about a week before they started wrapping their tiny fingers around mine, which was amazing. But the best bit was when Paul took his first steps walking to me. That was so exciting to see.

As they got a bit older, they got funnier too. One of the funniest things they ever did was rampaging around the kitchen with their walker. Chris was always fighting with it, and they'd crash around like mad.

The best thing about being a big sister to twins is how happy they are to see me. Sometimes they smile or laugh at me for no reason, and it makes me feel happy. They can be cheeky and mischievous, which isn't always my favourite thing, but it can be funny too.

The hardest thing is car journeys. I don't know why, but car journeys always make the crying worse, and that is definitely the worst sort of crying. Smelly nappies are bad too, but car crying is worse.

If the twins could talk, I think they'd say, "We are your brothers and we are very adorable." Or "We really like food. Would you like this carrot? Actually no, I've changed my mind. You can't have it." Paul would definitely talk about food all the time. Chris might talk about how good I am, or he might run off before you could hear what he was saying.

I'm proud of having twins. At first, I was shocked there were two of them, but now I just feel proud. Sometimes it's annoying when people get so excited about the twins that they forget about me. It feels like the twins have taken over the house and there's just so much stuff everywhere. I get used to it, but sometimes I think about what it was like before and how quiet it was. For quiet time now I enjoy drawing and Lego. I am even writing my own book about magical creatures.

Even with all that noise and mess, I wouldn't change having twin brothers. Holidays with them are my favourite, and when I come back from my dad's house, I'm always excited to see them. I don't have a favourite twin, because they're both so different and both so much fun in their own ways.

I don't think the cats like them at all. The boys don't stroke them nicely, they just grab their tails and yank on their fur. You'd think Timmy would run off, but she doesn't. She just stays there, hissing and glaring like it's all our fault while thinking "look at these little maggots".

Sometimes it feels like they've taken over the house, and it's easy to miss how quiet things used to be. But then I remember how boring it would be without them - Probably. They've made everything busier and louder, but also happier. And when they look up at me and laugh just because I'm there, it makes me feel like being their big sister is the best job in the world.

Double the stuff: choosing for two

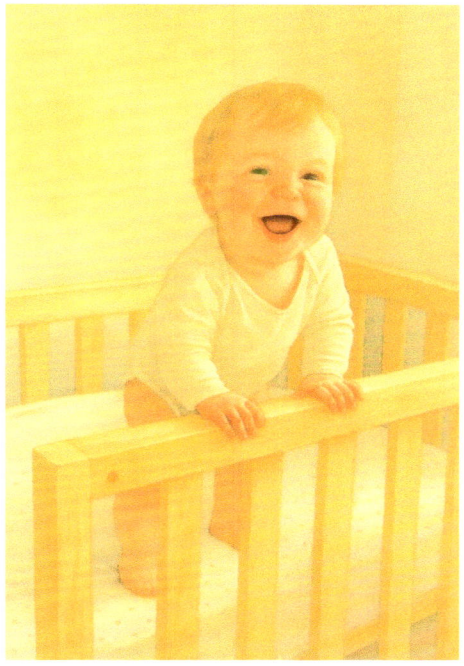

One of the biggest shocks with twins is just how much stuff you suddenly need. It's not just nappies and clothes, everything doubled, from cots to car seats, high chairs to bouncers. Not only the cost, but also the sheer number of decisions to make pose a challenge. Do you really need that miracle gadget? Will this buggy fit through your door? Does that monitor genuinely make life easier, or just add more stress?

We certainly didn't try every product out there, but we looked at a lot, and along the way learned what mattered for us and what didn't. Here's our take on some of the main dilemmas.

Cots: At first, we only had one cot because space in our modest house was tight. That worked fine until Chris, our little adventurer, started waking Paul up with his antics. Paul was *not* impressed. We quickly learned that separate yet connected beds were essential for everyone's sleep.

Instead of two cots, we went for toddler floor beds based on their slightly smaller footprint when two were side by side. The thinking for floorbeds was simple: if they managed to escape (and Chris certainly tried), at least it wasn't a big fall. Even now, the boys sometimes wake each other at 3 am, often with one deliberately squawking in the hope the other will join in, but having their own beds definitely helps. We also thought it might be easier on our backs than lowering babies into deep sided cots.

Buggies: One of the first big decisions we had to make was whether to go for a side-by-side buggy or one with the seats stacked. We were fortunate that our front door could accommodate a Bugaboo Donkey, and in the end we went with this option. It gives great flexibility, with seats that can face forwards, backwards, or even opposite directions, which makes outings much easier. It also handles really well compared to some of the top-heavy double-stack options, although it is heavy and not the most compact. During the summer the boys would get so hot and sweaty so we bought hoods with far more mesh. This made a huge difference and kept them cooler and happier.

The Bugaboo has been perfect in almost every way – smooth ride, comfy, easy to push. It does have its Achilles' heels. Lifts, for example, are definitely not its strong suit. When I take the twins to the university for meetings, they can't fit in the lift, a minor logistical nightmare.

Emma's birthday party at Ninja Warrior was another adventure. The buggy had to be completely dismantled and reassembled to navigate the venue's lifts, stairs and ramps. One of us would send the buggy up while the other wrangled the twins to the top, then we'd reassemble it midair like some kind of parent-engineering team. By the end, I found myself carrying both twins because it was simply the only way to get them in and out without creating full chaos.

It's a reminder that these larger, seemingly miraculous baby contraptions come with their own special set of challenges – and sometimes the only way forward is to improvise, sweat a bit, and try not to trip over your own feet while people look with a mixture of amusement and mild horror.

For everyday use the Donkey is excellent, but it's not always practical if you have a seven seater and lose space in the boot because of it. We were grateful to my sister for giving us their Out'n'About buggy as a lighter second option that folds much flatter, which is much easier for adventures, holidays, and when car boot space is tight.

A word of warning: buggies can be very expensive. While some can be picked up for a few hundred pounds new, once you add in bassinets and other essentials a new buggy can easily cost £1,500+. We kept an eye out for an affordable second hand option, when one came up we got it a bit sooner than perhaps we had liked (around week 23) but it saved us some money. All in with the modifications we still have probably spent £900.

So you don't get caught out later, make sure you measure your doorways and walk the routes you expect to use. If bins are always blocking the pavement or paths are narrow, you may want to consider a stacked option. The iCandy and Joie models, for example, can be configured with reversible seats, so the babies can face you or face forwards.

One final tip: if you look after your buggy well, you'll often be able to sell it on afterwards and recoup some of the cost.

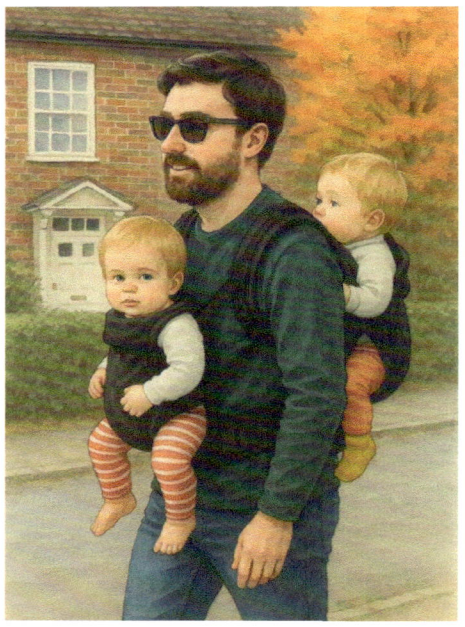

Slings and baby carriers: We had endless debates about slings and carriers, which brand to go for and what types we needed. In the end we went for two options that offered more versatility than a fabric sling in the longer term.

The Ergobaby 360 was brilliant from the early months onwards. The babies could face inward (a lifesaver in the middle of a nap battle), outward to watch the world go by, or be carried on the front or back. The boys loved it, and it became a go-to for shorter trips or sensory outings where the boys could explore places such as an arboretum. The downside is that it needs clipping at the back, which I could never quite manage by myself, though Cath is more flexible and could do it easily.

For longer walks, we spent more than we originally planned on a structured carrier, the LittleLife Freedom S4. It came with a built-in sunshade and proper back support, which made a huge difference. Trust us, as parents of twins, you really need to look after your back.

We also tried a twin sling (the Weego). It seemed a great idea, but by the time Cath was realistically able to use it the boys were already too big and we found it was hard on our backs when they got a lot bigger. For some parents it could be a real game-changer, though. We were given a TwinGo original which meant we can have one twin on the front and one for the back and can be used until the boys are 20kg.

Top tip: think about how you'll actually use each carrier day to day. Some are brilliant indoors or for popping out quickly, while others are designed for long walks. Having a mix gave us flexibility, and as importantly, gave our backs a bit of a break.

Remember aside from a twin carrier you will need two (obviously) which makes it harder if you are looking after them by yourself, sometimes though one of us went sling for one and buggy for the second.

Monitors: We didn't realise quite how many options there are for baby monitors, and the range of features is staggering. Some now come with sleep socks and other tracking add-ons. Honestly, we couldn't think of anything worse at home. We had those in hospital, and all they would have told us is what we already knew, our babies sleep awfully! We certainly didn't need a £400 system like the Dream Duo Sock & Cam 2 to remind us of that. Chris was even kicked off the sleep study at the hospital as his rubbish sleep didn't meet the minimum criteria.

Our main monitor is a VTech model, which we went for after a strong recommendation from a close friend. It's been reliable and easy to use, and we wouldn't be without it. We also bought a Badabulle Baby Online 300m Audio Monitor with a built-in night light for camping trips. It had good reviews and, most importantly, the range was far better than many others on the market, ideal for when we were outdoors.

Top tip: think about what you'll actually use. Features sound appealing on paper, but many just add cost without adding much real benefit. A good audio or video monitor with decent range, battery life, and reliability is far more valuable than something packed with gimmicks.

Car seats and cars: The boys hate their car seats, but we're glad we chose ones that spin. It helps protect our backs, which is a regular concern for parents of twins. In the early days car seats that could clip onto the Donkey buggy were useful for mid-nap transfers. Many families discover that their car isn't big enough once twins arrive. We couldn't afford a large seven-seater with a big boot, so we opted for a more affordable model and added a substantial roof box. This allows us to carry everything we need, buggy, car seats, luggage, and more.

Feeding cushions: One of the bits of kit we hadn't really thought much about before the boys arrived was feeding cushions. With twins, you suddenly discover there are dozens of options: some shaped for the rugby-ball hold (both babies tucked under your arms like you're about to make a break for the try line), others more traditional C- or V-shapes that sit across your lap like a double breakfast bar, and even wedge-style designs that look like something from a climbing gym.

At first, we thought we could make do with normal pillows. That fantasy lasted about five minutes. Standard cushions either slid away at the worst moment or collapsed under the weight of two hungry babies, leaving us contorted like amateur acrobats while trying to keep boobs and/or bottles in place.

In the end, we went for a Piglet cushion, and it turned out to be a brilliant choice, not just for the boys but for Cath as well. The extra back cushion was a lifesaver during those endless cluster feeds. It gave the twins plenty of space, stopped us feeling like we were stacking them like carry-on luggage, and saved Cath's back from giving up entirely. The only reason we used it less as time went on was reflux: the boys needed to be kept more upright, and the cushion held them flat. Even so, it became one of those essential items we relied on every single day in the early months. Again, a second hand Piglet with a spare cover saved us a lot of money.

High chairs and bibs: We have a range of bibs, including the ones that strap at the bottom to cover a high chair table by Bibado, the boys have discovered they can flick that strap back and forth while eating, just for fun. We have eight of these and it is still not enough as it only is enough for one day and the following breakfast. We would suggest keeping an eye out for these in the sale and getting more than you think you need.

For months our go to was the bib by Tidytot that looks like a UFO, unfortunately they've worked out that if you lift one side, the food catapults off beautifully. They may have been encouraged in this by Nana, who laughed the first time it happened. Ever since, they've treated it as a performance art. It probably is quite fun… unless you're one of our cats, who now live in fear of being splattered with half-chewed food. Because of the pinging, we can't use them anymore.

We've somehow ended up with a whole range of high chairs. There are a couple of IKEA ones that live in the garden or get dragged out onto the green, the trusty Stokke Tripp Trapps for the house, and for a while we even had two neat folding chairs that looked a bit like camping kit. The boys were never really comfortable in those, they always seemed to slump sideways like tiny drunks at a festival.

Don't believe the hype: There's an enormous amount of marketing aimed at new parents, each claiming their product will change your life, make your babies sleep, or make feeding easier. The truth is, there rarely is a miracle product, and what works for one family may do nothing for another. We've learned to take the claims with a pinch of salt and focus on what actually makes life manageable for us. One exception has been the Rockit rocker. It genuinely helps the boys stay asleep in their buggy for longer by replicating natural movement.

Lessons learned: In the early years, every extra item seems essential, but experience shows that some purchases aren't used as much as expected. Conversely, investing in versatile, well-made items (like the Donkey buggy or quality cots) can pay off long-term. Over time, you learn which items hold their value well if cared for, meaning you might recoup some of the cost when the children outgrow them.

Finances and budgeting

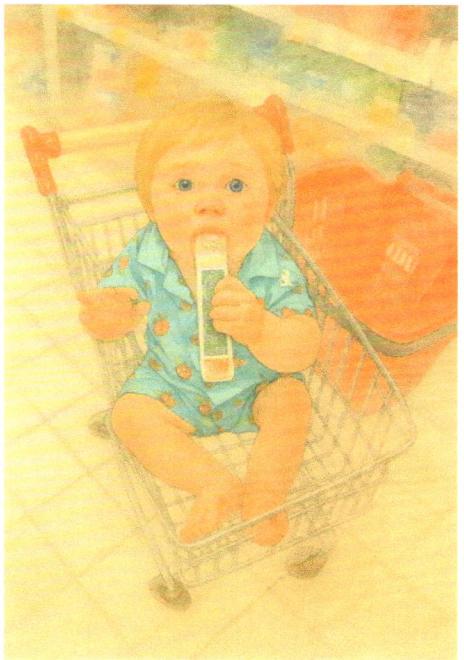

Twins don't just double the joy, they start off by doubling the cost... and then quietly triple it when you're not looking. Nappies, wipes, laundry detergent, these items all vanish at a suspiciously fast rate, as if the boys are running a black-market operation out of the changing bag. Add in rising mortgage rates, the cost-of-living crisis, and the quirks of heating a draughty 1930s house, and managing money feels like a hobby we never signed up for.

Some costs are obvious: two babies, two of everything. Others sneak up on you. Buggies, for example, apparently cost about the same as a second-hand car. Even second-hand, once you've added bassinets, rain covers, and coffee cup holders (trust us this is an essential rather than optional extra), the bill can easily creep into four figures. On the plus side, if you manage not to crash it into every doorway (unlike us), you might even sell it on later.

Then there's food. For a while, we were "just popping to the shop" every other day, and the receipts mounted faster than the laundry pile after a reflux incident. Now, we attempt a weekly shop and batch cook where we can, even if it means writing out a meal plan at 5:30 a.m. while refereeing a bout of Twin Wrestling during a late night feed. It's hardly glamorous, but it does keep the budget in check.

From the beginning, we set up a little "twin fund": £25 each a month, squirrelled away long before the boys even arrived. It's been a lifesaver for those inevitable surprises, like emergency osteopath trips, or when one twin suddenly needs a piece of kit that somehow costs more than our monthly food shop. Looking further ahead, we've even started pensions for them. Yes, they're still in nappies, but by the time they're 60, they'll be grateful for the miracle of compound interest.

Childcare was another financial awakening. We were incredibly lucky that just before the boys started nursery, the recently-introduced free hours eligible from 9-months increased from 15 to 30. Brilliant in theory, though the admin involved makes you wonder if the government secretly enjoys testing sleep-deprived parents' stamina. Even with free hours, there are extras. Meals cost £6 a day per child. Not outrageous but given Paul's love of discovering new food, they might have to charge us double.

Child benefit also chips in to help us a little. For twins, it's about £138 a month. Not a fortune, but enough to cover nappies, wipes, and maybe even a treat that isn't from the "reflux sale rail" at the supermarket. Combined with Tax Free Childcare where the government tops up some of what you put it, these small amounts really do add up.

We've also thought about the long game. Alongside the pensions, we put £25 a month each into a junior ISA and a bare trust. The ISA is untouchable until they're 18, while the bare trust gives us flexibility, so one day it might fund driving lessons, a school trip, or the insurance premium for when Twin Wrestling Productions moves from the cot to the car.

Then there are the quiet, creeping costs that no one warns you about. Shoes, for example. We knew they'd grow fast, but not this fast. Blink, and they've outgrown another pair,and of course, you can't just buy one set. By the time we'd worked out how to measure little feet properly, we'd practically bought shares in Clarks. Multiply everything by two, and suddenly even "basics" feel like a luxury line.

Hand-me-downs and freebies have been our saving grace. Friends, family, and the odd stranger from the local Facebook group have saved us hundreds, if not thousands. The twins don't care if the bouncer is a little scuffed or the jumper has a faded dinosaur print, and frankly, neither do we. We've ended up with a stash of gear that looks like the aftermath of a baby store clearance sale: two travel cots, three highchairs, and an absurd number of vests in every shade of beige imaginable.

Tom and Peter kindly passed down a range of their old toys that the boys play with all the time, including a little squishy man whose head squeaks when you press it. It has since become one of Paul's absolute favourites, to the point where he's often seen happily gnawing on it. We've named it "Cani-Paul," because apparently every beloved toy deserves a slightly odd family nickname.

The truth is, twins force you to think differently about money. Yes, it's easy to overspend, and yes, sometimes it feels like every direct debit in the country is addressed personally to us. But planning ahead, building small safety nets, and laughing at the absurdity helps. If you're struggling, the best thing you can do is talk about it. Whispering "we're fine" while secretly panic-Googling "grants for twin parents" at 2 a.m. doesn't help anyone.

Twin hacks & honest truths: what we wish we'd known

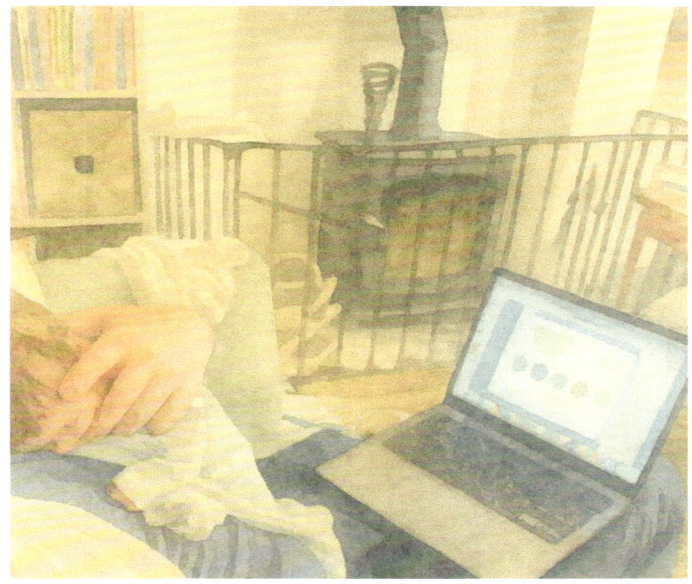

If we could go back to that first chaotic day, after one had just wee'd on their own face, we'd give ourselves a hug, a cup of tea, and a notepad. Surviving those first months with twins is like juggling flaming torches while riding a unicycle... blindfolded. Some of it's hilarious in hindsight, some soul-destroying at the time, and most of it involves vomit. Lots of vomit. There were nights where an hour of effort to get them to drink ended with vomit running down my back, and days where a single nap felt like winning the lottery.

Twins have a wicked sense of timing. They conspire to wake at the same moment, vomit in sync, or have a duet of screaming fits while you desperately try to work out whether the problem is milk, poo, reflux, or just the existential horror of life.

Exploding nappies? Guaranteed. Reflux? You'll become intimately familiar with its late-night trauma. Sleep? Forget it. Even the most well-planned routine can end with you clutching a bottle, a muslin, and your sanity in tatters. And yes, there were sympathetic looks from strangers in Burley in the New Forest when our distracted boys staged their public feeding disasters, it's funny now, but hard at the time.

Our Most Useful Hacks

Sleep in bits, not blocks: Twenty minutes in the middle of the day is gold if it is all you have.

Tandem feeding is intense but magical: A big scarf, a piglet pillow, and some creative contortions are lifesavers.

Bottles can be a relief: Changing one evening feed from breastfeeding to a bottle around 7pm took some pressure off Cath.

Gear is optional, but plan ahead: Keep an eye out for second-hand buggies and equipment your bank balance will thank you.

Celebrate tiny wins: A nap longer than 30 minutes, a full feed, a smile at the right moment. These little things are all victories.

Ask for help: Even 20 minutes of someone holding a baby while you shower or breathe is miraculous.

Music can be a secret weapon: We tried Bridgerton instead of white noise, sometimes the harps and flutes helped, sometimes not, but it was worth a try.

Vomit and nappies are part of the package: Accept it, laugh about it later, and keep many muslins handy.

Trust Your Instincts: Forget unsolicited advice. What worked for a single baby decades ago will probably fail spectacularly with two. People will comment, people will judge, but you know your twins best. Trust your instincts, and don't be scared to ask for help when needed. The despair of trying to get milk into them, only for it to come straight back out, is real. You will survive it and probably laugh about it one day.

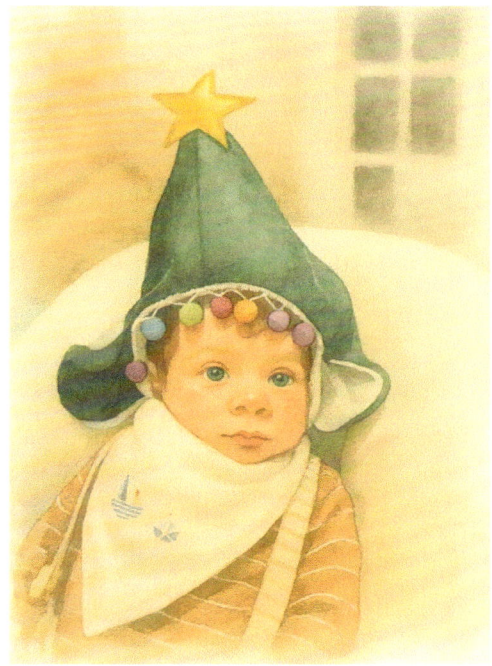

Hold Onto the Memories: Amid the chaos, there are moments of pure joy that are easy to forget when sleep deprived: Paul's first crab-inspired steps, Chris being a little festive Christmas tree, the terror of leaves falling on a face, the cries that sound like tweeting birds, the fear in the cats' eyes when a plum comes flying during feeding time at the zoo, and the smiles from two beautiful boys. The look Emma gave when she first held them is a memory we'll never forget and Cath's expression watching Paul walk on the green is another keeper. Laugh at the chaos, forgive yourself for the disasters, and celebrate the tiny victories. These are the treasures.

By writing this, I've realised there are certain little things they used to do that I really loved, but just don't happen anymore. Having two tiny babies on my shoulders while writing for example. Or when you'd walk with a sling and have a little boy tucked in, if you put your finger near him, he'd instinctively grab it and give it a gentle hold. Those tiny, innate gestures are a distant memory. I guess that's the difference time makes, but it's a reminder that all these small, precious moments don't last forever.

What we'd say to someone starting their twin journey

Brace yourself for unpredictability, keep your sense of humour, and stock up on muslins. Plan, but don't be paralysed by planning. Trust your instincts, ask for help, and hold onto the moments of joy, they come faster than you think. Chaos is temporary, but the memories last forever (especially if you write them in a book!).

Epilogue – Surviving year one, birthdays and outsourcing the mayhem to nursery

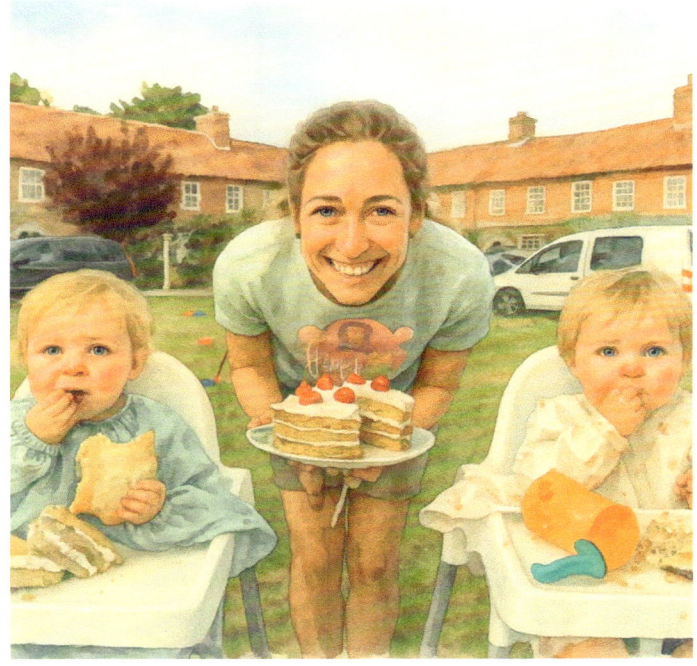

The first year has been a rollercoaster of triumphs, disasters, and a lot of sleepless nights we will pretend we do not remember. Just when we thought we were mastering the juggle, along came birthday candles, cake-covered chaos, and the first tentative steps into nursery life.

Genuinely, I thought that with less than one week to go until their first birthday the chaos might finally start to subside. Instead, more happened in a few days than you would think possible. We had practically finished writing this book by then and even sent it off for proofing, but clearly life had not read the deadline and decided to throw in a few bonus chapters for good measure.

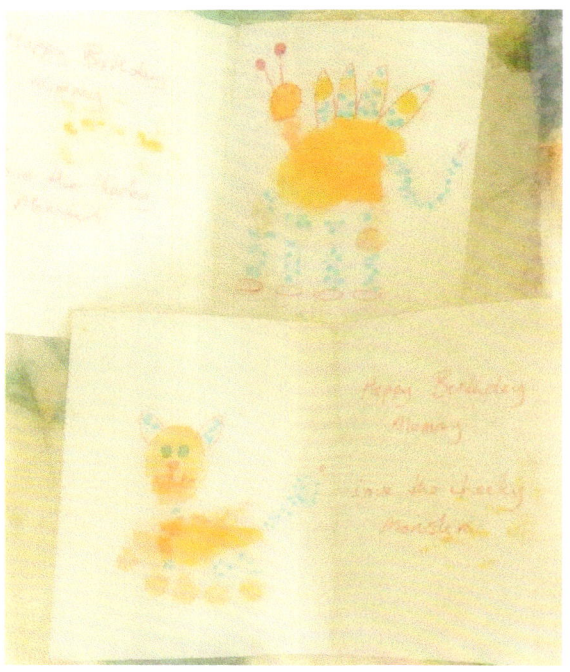

The first milestone was Cath's birthday. It was her first since the boys were born and I was determined to make it special. They, of course, had other ideas. The day before, I had attempted the classic "cute baby handprint card" where their palms became a cupcake with candles and a balloon. We had been to The Makers House in Fareham a few times to decorate pottery and they made it look so simple. At home, it was chaos. I tried their feet instead and had a little more success, adapting the prints into cheeky little monsters. The boys needed a full washdown afterwards as they were covered in ink, but at least the card had character.

Cath was working the morning of her birthday, and in true show-stealing style Chris chose that very moment to try walking when I took them for a romp on the Common. I scooped him up, much to his disgust, so we could surprise Cath at work. Luckily he forgave me and performed a wobbling, applause-filled stumble straight towards her, as if he had been saving the moment just for her birthday.

We had originally planned two gatherings that week, one for Cath and one for the boys, both on the green outside our house. The Great British weather had other ideas. With rain threatening, we combined both parties on the 9th, Cath's birthday, which meant she had to share her celebration with two nearly one-year-olds who cared far more about ripping paper than opening presents. It still felt like an achievement worth raising a glass to. It also led to some very confused singing of Happy Birthday, no one could quite decide who they were addressing.

Of course, life is never all cake and bunting. In the middle of a routine trip to Sainsbury's, Paul went blue and passed out. A well-meaning bystander rang 999 before I could explain that this was something we had been dealing with since he was six weeks old. The call handler insisted we needed to be in A&E within the hour. So instead of attending their first birthday party, I called Cath and we spent the afternoon in hospital. The boys thought it was brilliant. Paul in particular was fascinated by the sliding glass doors, happily bashing on them and grinning at everyone who passed, while Cath and I quietly despaired. The NHS staff were brilliant, full checks and a 12-lead ECG later, both boys were given the all-clear. Though the doctor's comment that "this might carry on until they are five or six" nearly broke me.

The only consolation was being handed iron supplements. I had always thought of iron as something to stop you looking pale and tired, but it turns out it's also crucial for carrying oxygen and helping the brain regulate breathing. Without enough of it, the system gets a bit jumpy: a small upset can trip the wiring when breathing pauses, suddenly colour drains, and parents panic. Once we understood that, the supplements made a lot more sense, even if they came with the bonus of nappies best described as "experimental art projects."

That week also brought a different kind of breakthrough. Our friend Ping, an audiologist, helped us finally work out what was happening with Paul's hearing. While we waited for a referral for fitting hearing aids, Ping suggested trying headphones and a microphone. It took some creative fiddling to fit a wriggly one-year-old, but the effect was instant. For the first time, Paul reacted to quiet noises without us having to shout, wave or clap like over-enthusiastic seals. The grin on his face was unforgettable, pure joy at hearing the world properly. If only he would agree to keep the headphones on for more than a few minutes, we might be able to read him a whole story.

On the morning of their actual birthday, the boys decided the best way to celebrate was to remind us exactly how terrible they are at sleeping. Cath nudged me awake at 2.30am in need of help. "Which one have I got?" I mumbled. "I don't know!" she replied. Two hours later both boys were still wide-eyed, chatting away like they were hosting an afterparty. I had paced, rocked, and shushed so much that my watch congratulated me for hitting my step count before sunrise. Perhaps from now on their birthday gift to us could be a proper night's sleep. Although knowing them, we will probably get another round of midnight mischief instead.

Later that day, on the walk to a friend of theirs birthday party, they were in full performance mode, clapping at everything: birds, trees, people, even some very confused dogs. Clearly the disturbed night had left its mark on us more than on them. On the way home, still buzzing, they reached out from their seats and clasped hands, giggling through their own private game of peekaboo. Then Chris, never one to miss a spotlight moment, lunged dramatically at Paul's face like a pint-sized gladiator. Paul thought it was the funniest thing he'd ever seen, and the pair dissolved into helpless giggles.

The party itself had a very special guest: Lisa from Hartbeeps, who the boys absolutely adore from their Thursday sessions (sadly a thing of the past since Cath's return to work). Her arrival meant familiar songs and games that we have got used to singing at home and also a chance for the boys to show off their "moves" and meet lots of new little buddies. Best of all, there was a ball pool, which both boys launched into like tiny Olympians and refused to get out of.

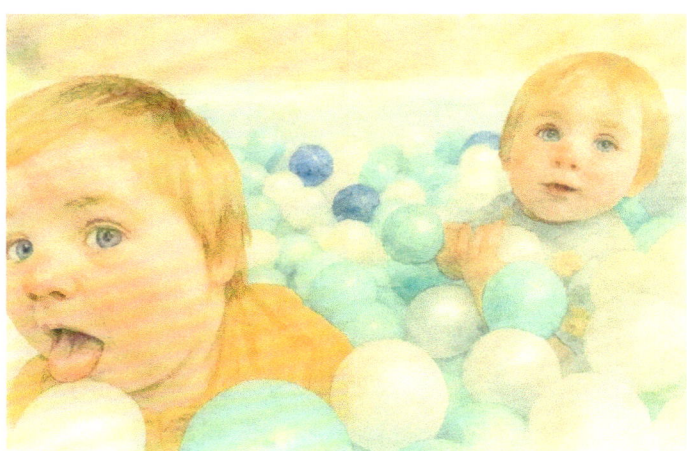

Later, we headed to Nana and Papa's to celebrate with family. As expected, the biggest hits of the day were not the presents but the tape, the boxes and the wrapping paper. We got some amazing books about bees, frogs, dinosaurs, goblins and bears. Next door had given a book about animals eating snacks, which Paul latched onto instantly. Chris, true to form, was far more taken with the book about farts.

Dinner brought its own entertainment. Each boy had a helium balloon, which they clutched like prized possessions, utterly entranced. The cake was topped with a rocket candle that showered sparks dramatically into the air. We had bought it specifically to avoid the stress of persuading two one-year-olds to blow out a flame. We have seen too many toddlers reach gleefully towards lit candles.

The following week came another milestone: nursery. The boys started two days a week, with a few settling-in sessions first. Paul instantly bonded with a plastic chicken leg (proof that snacks are life), while Chris discovered a plastic fish almost as tall as he was and the magic of soft play. The twins have a brilliant key worker, who, as fate would have it, also has two black cats. When I showed the boys her photo on the wall, Paul pointed with his trusty Peter Pointer and proudly signed "cat," as if to say, "We approve."

Starting nursery also meant the end of Daddy Day Care three days a week. I loved it, but my goodness it was exhausting. Nursery feels like a proper turning point, a chance for the boys to explore the world beyond our four walls, and for us to finally drink a cup of coffee while it is still hot. Somehow it feels like both the end of an era and the start of a brand new adventure. Yet we are still standing, or at least mostly upright.

The next year will no doubt bring more of the same in some ways: nappies, noise, and endless laundry. But there will also be new milestones, with the biggest on the horizon being Chris walking properly. That will open up a whole new level of chaos, that even Paul's crab-walk beginnings could not prepare us for.

For Cath and me, the end of the first year is bittersweet. We are enormously proud to have survived the hardest, messiest, most sleep-deprived twelve months of our lives, but also a little sad at how quickly it has all changed. Those tiny moments, the way they instinctively grabbed a finger in the sling, how they slept with their bums stuck in the air, or how their cries once sounded like tweeting birds, are already slipping into memory.

Then there is Emma. Watching her become a big sister this year has been a joy in itself. From the look she gave when she first held the twins to the way she has learned to share her space, her patience, and even her cheekiness, she has grown just as much as the boys have. She is eight going on eighteen, full of opinions and eye-rolls, but also full of kindness. This year has asked a lot of her, with new responsibilities, less attention, and the general chaos that comes with two brothers. She has had to build her own kind of resilience, becoming a little more self-sufficient and a lot more sure of herself. We could not be prouder.

So here we are at the end of year one. Two toddlers, one brilliant big sister, two tired parents, and a family that somehow keeps laughing even when it all goes wrong. Whatever the next year holds, we'll muddle through together. If nothing else, we know it will never be boring.

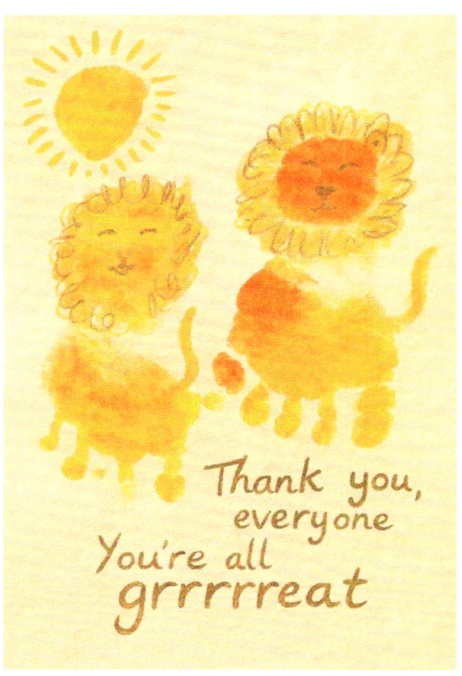

Thank you,
everyone
You're all
grrrrreat

We would like to thank everyone at Princess Anne Hospital who supported us throughout this journey, from the specialist midwives to the incredible staff who cared for us during every appointment, scan, and stay. Your kindness, patience, and expertise made an overwhelming experience so much easier to navigate, and we will always be grateful. Without you, we wouldn't have two wonderful boys brightening every day of our lives.

A special thank you also goes to the team at the AMSDEC unit in Ipswich for their guidance and support, especially when Dave and Dave-Dave gave us a scare while we were on holiday. Knowing we had your knowledge and reassurance behind us at every stage was an incredible comfort, and we could not have done it without you.

We are endlessly grateful to everyone who has supported us through the chaos, the sleepless nights, and the full-scale poopocalypses. Far too many to list individually, and let's be honest, it's probably a good job we haven't tried, because we can barely remember anything anymore. We are truly grateful to you all.

A special shout-out goes to the Heathers, the Salters, the Thompsons, the Wynne-Joneses, the Atcherleys, the Waites, the Frasers, the Hamilton-Bartletts (but not you Ed) as well as others such as Kris, Mehtap, and both of our families for always stepping in with practical help, advice, or just a sympathetic ear when it all felt a bit much. Some new friends have come out of this journey, particularly the Everetts. Thanks as well to the various colleagues who have also helped us cope with this new transition and with work. Thanks to Sian for returning from Fiji laden with presents for baby cuddles and curry! Jess, Claire, Emma and Kirsty deserve a special mention here, since Jess was the person who suggested this book in the first place.

Thanks also to everyone who contributed to the food train set up by Jude which was extended multiple times, sent gifts for the boys (and sometimes for Cath), or simply checked in to remind us that we weren't alone in surviving twin life. You've made an enormous difference.

The Wells Road Mamas, the Wet Animals and the Length deserve a special mention for looking after Cath remotely and coming down to help her when we came back from hospital.

We're particularly grateful to Paul Booth for proofing the first draft. Usually he helps me with archaeological work rather than twin memoirs! Cath would also like to thank the editor of the Clausentum Press for putting up with Richard.

Enormous thanks to our families (parents, siblings, cousins) for their unwavering support and, of course, Emma, who has been our constant source of joy, perspective, and sanity (well, some of the time).

Finally, thank you for buying this book and helping support the outstanding neonatal care in Southampton.

BV - #0140 - 201025 - C46 - 229/152/9 - PB - 9781919242705 - Gloss Lamination